Statistics at Square One

This book is to be returned on or before the last date stamped below.

2 5 APR 2013

2 2 MAY 2013
0 2 APR 2014

This edition first published 2009, © 2009 by M.J. Campbell and T.D.V. Swinscow
Previous editions: 1976, 1977, 1978, 1978, 1979, 1980, 1980, 1983, 1996, 2002

BMJ Books is an imprint of BMJ Publishing Group Limited, used under licence by Blackwell Publishing
which was acquired by John Wiley & Sons in February 2007. Blackwell's publishing programme has
been merged with Wiley's global Scientific, Technical and Medical business to form Wiley-Blackwell.

Registered office: John Wiley & Sons Ltd, The Atrium, Southern Gate, Chichester, West Sussex,
PO19 8SQ, UK

Editorial offices: 9600 Garsington Road, Oxford, OX4 2DQ, UK
The Atrium, Southern Gate, Chichester, West Sussex, PO19 8SQ, UK
111 River Street, Hoboken, NJ 07030-5774, USA

For details of our global editorial offices, for customer services and for information about how
to apply for permission to reuse the copyright material in this book please see our website at
www.wiley.com/wiley-blackwell

The right of the author to be identified as the author of this work has been asserted in accordance
with the Copyright, Designs and Patents Act 1988.

Wiley also publishes its books in a variety of electronic formats. Some content that appears in print
may not be available in electronic books.

Designations used by companies to distinguish their products are often claimed as trademarks.
All brand names and product names used in this book are trade names, service marks, trademarks
or registered trademarks of their respective owners. The publisher is not associated with any product
or vendor mentioned in this book. This publication is designed to provide accurate and authoritative
information in regard to the subject matter covered. It is sold on the understanding that the publisher
is not engaged in rendering professional services. If professional advice or other expert assistance is
required, the services of a competent professional should be sought.

The contents of this work are intended to further general scientific research, understanding, and
discussion only and are not intended and should not be relied upon as recommending or promoting
a specific method, diagnosis, or treatment by physicians for any particular patient. The publisher and
the author make no representations or warranties with respect to the accuracy or completeness of the
contents of this work and specifically disclaim all warranties, including without limitation any implied
warranties of fitness for a particular purpose. In view of ongoing research, equipment modifications,
changes in governmental regulations, and the constant flow of information relating to the use of
medicines, equipment, and devices, the reader is urged to review and evaluate the information
provided in the package insert or instructions for each medicine, equipment, or device for, among
other things, any changes in the instructions or indication of usage and for added warnings and
precautions. Readers should consult with a specialist where appropriate. The fact that an organization
or Website is referred to in this work as a citation and/or a potential source of further information
does not mean that the author or the publisher endorses the information the organization or Website
may provide or recommendations it may make. Further, readers should be aware that Internet
Websites listed in this work may have changed or disappeared between when this work was written
and when it is read. No warranty may be created or extended by any promotional statements for this
work. Neither the publisher nor the author shall be liable for any damages arising herefrom.

Library of Congress Cataloging-in-Publication Data

Campbell, Michael J., PhD.
Statistics at square one/M.J. Campbell and T.D.V. Swinscow.—11th ed.
p. ; cm.
Includes bibliographical references and index.
ISBN 978-1-4051-9100-5
1. Medical statistics. 2. Statistics. I. Swinscow, T. D. V. (Thomas Douglas Victor) II. Title.
[DNLM: 1. Statistics as Topic. WA 950 C189s 2009]
RA407.C355 2009
610.72—dc22

2009003028

ISBN: 978-1-4051-9100-5

A catalogue record for this book is available from the British Library.

Set in 9.25/12pt Meridien by Macmillan Publishing Solutions, Chennai, India
Printed in Singapore

3   2010

CHAPTER 1
Data display and summary

Types of data

The first step, before any calculations or plotting of data, is to decide what type of data one is dealing with. There are a number of typologies, but one that has proven useful is given in Table 1.1. The basic distinction is between quantitative variables (for which one asks "how much?") and categorical variables (for which one asks "what type?").

Quantitative variables can either be *measured* or *counted*. Measured variables, such as height, can in theory take any value within a given range and are termed *continuous*. However, even continuous variables can only be measured to a certain degree of

Table 1.1 Examples of types of data.

Quantitative	
Measured	Counted
Blood pressure, height, weight, age	Number of children in a family
	Number of attacks of asthma per week
	Number of cases of AIDS in a city
Categorical	
Ordinal (ordered categories)	Nominal (unordered categories)
Grade of breast cancer	Sex (male/female)
Better, same, worse	Alive or dead
Disagree, neutral, agree	Blood group O, A, B, AB

Statistics at Square One, XIth edition. By M.J. Campbell and T.D.V. Swinscow. Published 2009 by Blackwell Publishing, ISBN: 9781405191005.

accuracy. Thus, age is often measured in years, height in centimeters. Examples of crude measured variables would be shoe or hat sizes, which only take a limited range of values. Counted variables are counts with a given time or area. Examples of counted variables are number of children in a family and number of attacks of asthma per week.

Categorical variables are either nominal (unordered) or ordinal (ordered). Nominal variables with just two levels are often termed *binary*. Examples of binary variables are male/female, diseased/ not diseased, alive/dead. Variables with more than two categories where the order does not matter are also termed *nominal*, such as blood group O, A, B, AB. These are not ordered since one cannot say that people in blood group B lie between those in A and those in AB. Sometimes, however, the categories can be ordered, and the variable is termed *ordinal*. Examples include grade of breast cancer, or a Likert scale where people can "agree", "neither agree nor disagree", or "disagree" with some statement. In this case, the order does matter and it is usually important to account for it.

Variables shown in the top section of Table 1.1 can be converted to ones below by using "cut-off points". For example, blood pressure can be turned into a nominal variable by defining "hypertension" as a diastolic blood pressure greater than 90 mmHg, and "normotension" as blood pressure less than or equal to 90 mmHg. Height (continuous) can be converted into "short", "average", or "tall" (ordinal). In general, it is easier to summarize categorical variables, and so quantitative variables are often converted to categorical ones for descriptive purposes. To make a clinical decision about a patient, one does not need to know the exact serum potassium level (continuous) but whether it is within the normal range (nominal). It may be easier to think of the proportion of the population who are hypertensive than the distribution of blood pressure. However, categorizing a continuous variable reduces the amount of information available, and statistical tests will in general be more sensitive—that is, they will have more power (see Chapter 6 for a definition of power)—for a continuous variable than the corresponding nominal one, although more assumptions may have to be made about the data. Categorizing data is therefore useful for summarizing results, but not for statistical analysis. However, it is often not appreciated that the choice of appropriate cut-off points can be difficult, and different choices can lead to different conclusions about a set of data.

These definitions of types of data are not unique, nor are they mutually exclusive, and are given as an aid to help an investigator decide how to display and analyze data. Data which are effectively counts, such as death rates, are commonly analyzed as continuous if the disease is not rare. One should not debate overlong the typology of a particular variable!

Stem and leaf plots

Before any statistical calculation, even the simplest, is performed, the data should be tabulated or plotted. If they are quantitative and relatively few, say up to about 30, they are conveniently written down in order of size.

For example, a pediatric registrar in a district general hospital is investigating the amount of lead in the urine of children from a nearby housing estate. In a particular street, there are 15 children whose ages range from 1 year to under 16, and in a preliminary study the registrar has found the following amounts of urinary lead (μmol/24 h), given in Table 1.2.

Table 1.2 Urinary concentration of lead in 15 children from housing estate (μmol/24 h).

0.6, 2.6, 0.1, 1.1, 0.4, 2.0, 0.8, 1.3, 1.2, 1.5, 3.2, 1.7, 1.9, 1.9, 2.2

A simple way to order, and also to display, the data is to use a stem and leaf plot. To do this we need to abbreviate the observations to two significant digits. In the case of the urinary concentration data, the digit to the left of the decimal point is the "stem" and the digit to the right the "leaf".

We first write the stems in order down the page. We then work along the data set, writing the leaves down "as they come". Thus, for the first data point, we write a 6 opposite the 0 stem. These are as given in Figure 1.1.

Stem	Leaf						
0	6	1	4	8			
1	1	3	2	5	7	9	9
2	6	0	2				
3	2						

Figure 1.1 Stem and leaf "as they come".

Stem	Leaf						
0	1	4	6	8			
1	1	2	3	5	7	9	9
2	0	2	6				
3	2						

Figure 1.2 Ordered stem and leaf plot.

We then order the leaves, as in Figure 1.2.

The advantage of first setting the figures out in order of size and not simply feeding them straight from notes into a calculator (e.g. to find their mean) is that the relation of each to the next can be looked at. Is there a steady progression, a noteworthy hump, a considerable gap? Simple inspection can disclose irregularities. Furthermore, a glance at the figures gives information on their *range*. The smallest value is 0.1 and the largest is 3.2 μmol/24 h. Note that the range can mean two numbers (smallest, largest) or a single number (largest minus smallest). We will usually use the former when displaying data, but when talking about summary measures (see Chapter 2) we will think of the range as a single number.

Median

To find the median (or midpoint) we need to identify the point which has the property that half the data are greater than it, and half the data are less than it. For 15 points, the midpoint is clearly the eighth largest, so that seven points are less than the median and seven points are greater than it. This is easily obtained from Figure 1.2 by counting from the top to the eighth leaf, which is 1.50 μmol/24 h.

To find the median for an even number of points, the procedure is illustrated by an example.

Suppose the pediatric registrar obtained a further set of 16 urinary lead concentrations from children living in the countryside in the same county as the hospital (Table 1.3).

To obtain the median we average the eighth and ninth points (1.8 and 1.9) to get 1.85 μmol/24 h. In general, if n is even, we average the $(n/2)$th largest and the $(n/2 + 1)$th largest observations.

The main advantage of using the median as a measure of location is that it is "robust" to outliers. For example, if we had accidentally written 34 rather than 3.4 in Table 1.3, the median would

Table 1.3 Urinary concentration of lead in 16 rural children (μmol/24 h).

0.2, 0.3, 0.6, 0.7, 0.8, 1.5, 1.7, 1.8, 1.9, 1.9, 2.0, 2.0, 2.1, 2.8, 3.1, 3.4

still have been 1.85. One disadvantage is that it is tedious to order a large number of observations by hand (there is usually no "median" button on a calculator).

An interesting property of the median is shown by first subtracting the median from each observation, and changing the negative signs to positive ones (taking the absolute difference). For the data in Table 1.3, the median is 1.5 and the absolute differences are 0.9, 1.1, 1.4, 0.4, 1.1, 0.5, 0.7, 0.2, 0.3, 0.0, 1.7, 0.2, 0.4, 0.4, 0.7. The sum of these is 10.0. It can be shown that no other data point will give a smaller sum. Thus the median is the point "nearest" to all the other data points.

Measures of variation

It is informative to have some measure of the variation of observations about the median. A simple measure is the range, which is the difference between the maximum and minimum values (although in Statistics, it is usually given as two numbers: the minimum and the maximum). The range is very susceptible to what are known as *outliers*, points well outside the main body of the data. For example, if we had made the mistake of writing 32 instead 3.2 in Table 1.2, then the range would be written as 0.1 to 32 μmol/24 h, which is clearly misleading.

A more robust approach is to divide the distribution of the data into four, and find the points below which are 25%, 50%, and 75% of the distribution. These are known as *quartiles*, and the median is the second quartile. The variation of the data can be summarized in the interquartile range, the distance between the first and third quartile, often abbreviated to IQR. With small data sets, it may not be possible to divide the data set into exact quarters, and there are a variety of proposed methods to estimate the quartiles. One method is based on the fact that for n observations we can theoretically have values less than the smallest and greater than the largest, so if we order the observations there are $n - 1$ spaces between the observations, but $n + 1$ areas in total. Thus the 1st, 2nd, and 3rd quartiles are estimated by points which are the $(n + 1)/4$, $(n + 1)/2$, and

$3(n + 1)/4$ points. For 15 observations, these are the 4th, 8th, and 12th points and from Figure 1.2, we find the values 0.8 and 2.0 which gives the IQR. For 16 points, the quartiles correspond to the 4.25, 8.5, and 12.75th points. To estimate, say the lower quartile, we find the 4th and 5th points, and then find a value which is one quarter the distance from the 4th to the 5th. Thus the 4th and 5th points are 0.7 and 0.8, respectively, and we get $0.7 + 0.25(0.8 - 0.7) = 0.725$. For the upper quartile we want a point which is three quarters the distance from the 12th to the 13th points, 2.0 and 2.1, and we get $2.0 + 0.75 \times (2.1 - 2.0) = 2.075$. The median is the second quartile and is calculated as before. Thus the three quartiles are 0.725, 1.85, and 2.075.

An alternative method, known as Tukey's hinges, is to find the points which are themselves medians between each end of the range and the median. Thus, from Figure 1.2, there are eight points between and including the smallest, 0.1, and the median, 1.5. Thus the midpoint lies between 0.8 and 1.1, or 0.95. This is the first quartile. Similarly the third quartile is midway between 1.9 and 2.0, or 1.95. Thus, by this method, the IQR is 0.95 to 1.95 μmol/24 h. These values are given by OpenStat. For large data sets, the two methods will agree, but as one can see, for small data sets they may differ.

Data display

The simplest way to show data is a dot plot. Figure 1.3 shows the data from Tables 1.2 and 1.3 together with the median for each set. Take care if you use a scatterplot option in a computer program to plot these data: you may find the points with the same value are plotted on top of each other.

Sometimes the points in separate plots may be linked in some way; for example, the data in Tables 1.2 and 1.3 may result from a matched case–control study (see Chapter 13 for a description of this type of study) in which individuals from the countryside were matched by age and sex with individuals from the town. If possible the links should be maintained in the display, for example by joining matching individuals in Figure 1.3. This can lead to a more sensitive way of examining the data.

When the data sets are large, plotting individual points can be cumbersome. An alternative is a box–whisker plot. The box is marked by the first and third quartile, and the whiskers extend to the range. The median is also marked in the box, as shown in Figure 1.4.

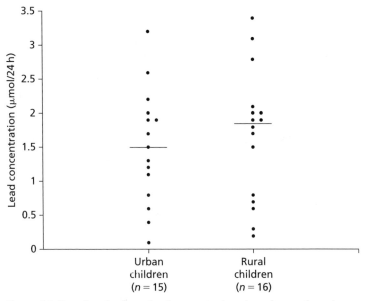

Figure 1.3 Dot plot of urinary lead concentrations for urban and rural children (with medians).

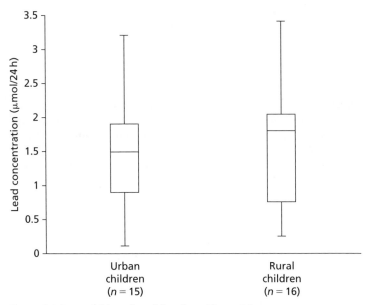

Figure 1.4 Box–whisker plot of data from Figure 1.3.

Table 1.4 Lead concentration in 140 urban children.

Lead concentration (μmol/24h)	Number of children
0–	2
0.4–	7
0.8–	10
1.2–	16
1.6–	23
2.0–	28
2.4–	19
2.8–	16
3.2–	11
3.6–	7
4.0–	1
4.4	
Total	140

It is easy to include more information in a box–whisker plot. One method, which is implemented in some computer programs, is to extend the whiskers only to points that are $Q_1 - 1.5 \times$ IQR to $Q_3 + 1.5 \times$ IQR, where Q_1 and Q_3 are the first (lower) and third (upper) quartiles, respectively, and to show remaining points as dots. This way, outlying points are shown separately.

Histograms

Suppose the pediatric registrar referred to earlier extends the urban study to the entire estate in which the children live. He obtains figures for the urinary lead concentration in 140 children aged over 1 year and under 16. We can display these data as a grouped frequency table (Table 1.4). These can also be displayed as a histogram as in Figure 1.5. Note one should always give the sample size on the histogram.

Bar charts

Suppose, of the 140 children, 20 lived in owner occupied houses, 70 lived in council houses, and 50 lived in private rented accommodation. Figures from the census suggest that for this age group, throughout the county, 50% live in owner occupied houses, 30%

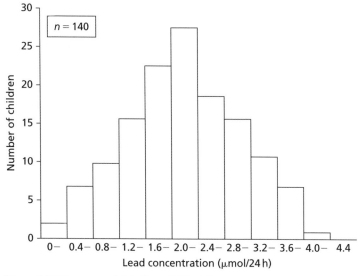

Figure 1.5 Histogram of data from Table 1.4.

in council houses, and 20% in private rented accommodation. Type of accommodation is a categorical variable, which can be displayed in a bar chart. We first express our data as percentages: 14% owner occupied, 50% council house, 36% private rented. We then display the data as a bar chart. The sample size should always be given (Figure 1.6).

Common questions

What is the distinction between a histogram and a bar chart?

Alas, with modern graphics programs, the distinction is often lost. A histogram shows the distribution of a continuous variable and, since the variable is continuous, there should be no gaps between the bars. A bar chart shows the distribution of a discrete variable or a categorical one, and so will have spaces between the bars. It is a mistake to use a bar chart to display a summary statistic such as a mean, particularly when it is accompanied by some measure of variation to produce a "dynamite plunger plot."[1] It is better to use a box–whisker plot.

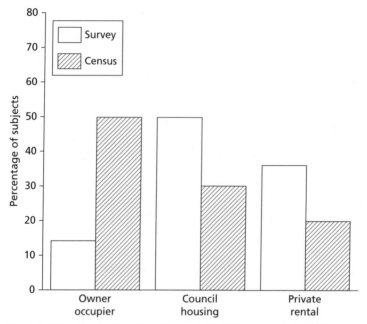

Figure 1.6 Bar chart of housing data for 140 children and comparable census data.

How many groups should I have for a histogram?

In general one should choose enough groups to show the shape of a distribution, but not too many to lose the shape in the noise. It is partly aesthetic judgement but, in general, between 5 and 15, depending on the sample size, gives a reasonable picture. Try to keep the intervals (known also as "bin widths") equal. With equal intervals, the height of the bars and the area of the bars are both proportional to the number of subjects in the group. With unequal intervals, this link is lost, and interpretation of the figure can be difficult.

Displaying data in papers

• The general principle should be, as far as possible, to show the original data and to try not to obscure the design of a study in the display. Within the constraints of legibility, show as much information as possible. Thus if a data set is small (say <20 points) a dot plot is preferred to a box–whisker plot.

- Note that the quartiles are *points* not areas, so one can say an observation is above the third quartile or in the top quarter, not in the top quartile. There are only three quartiles and four quarters.
- When displaying the relationship between two quantitative variables, use a scatterplot (Chapter 11) in preference to categorizing one or both of the variables.
- If data points are matched or from the same patient, link them with lines where possible.
- *Pie charts* are another way to display categorical data, but they are rarely better than a bar chart or a simple table.
- To compare the distribution of two or more data sets, it is often better to use box–whisker plots side by side than histograms. Another common technique is to treat the histograms as if they were bar charts, and plot the bars for each group adjacent to each other.
- When quoting a range or IQR, give the two numbers that define it, rather than the difference.
- The median and IQR should be given to the same accuracy as the original data or one extra significant digit if an average of two points is needed. Thus in Table 1.3, the original data are quoted to one decimal place and the median to two decimal places.

Exercises

1.1 From the 140 children whose urinary concentration of lead was investigated, 40 were chosen who were aged at least 1 year but under 5 years. The following concentrations of copper (in μmol/24 h) were found.

0.70, 0.45, 0.72, 0.30, 1.16, 0.69, 0.83, 0.74, 1.24, 0.77,
0.65, 0.76, 0.42, 0.94, 0.36, 0.98, 0.64, 0.90, 0.63, 0.55,
0.78, 0.10, 0.52, 0.42, 0.58, 0.62, 1.12, 0.86, 0.74, 1.04,
0.65, 0.66, 0.81, 0.48, 0.85, 0.75, 0.73, 0.50, 0.34, 0.88

    (a) Draw a stem and leaf plot and find the median, range, and quartiles.

    (b) Playing with the data: Change the value 1.24 to 2.24. See how the statistics found in (a) are affected. Change 0.36 to −0.36 and also look at the results.

1.2 A physician in an emergency room (ER) is collecting data. What sort of data are the following: Time in minutes waiting in ER, triage outcome (no injury, minor injury, major injury), number of cases of road accident victims in the ER, type of accident in the ER (fall, road accident, assault)?

Reference

1. Freeman JV, Walters SJ and Campbell MJ. *How to Display Data.* Oxford: Wiley-Blackwell, 2007.

CHAPTER 2

Summary statistics for quantitative data

Summary statistics summarize the essential information in a data set into a few numbers, which, for example, can be communicated verbally. The median and the interquartile range discussed in Chapter 1 are examples of summary statistics. Here we discuss summary statistics for quantitative data.

Mean and standard deviation

The median is known as a measure of location; that is, it tells us where the data are. As stated in Chapter 1, we do not need to know all the data values exactly to calculate the median; if we made the smallest value even smaller or the largest value even larger, it would not change the value of the median. Thus the median does not use all the information in the data and so it can be shown to be less efficient than the mean or average, which does use all values of the data. To calculate the mean, we add up the observed values and divide by their number. The total of the values obtained in Table 1.2 was 22.5 μmol/24 h, which was divided by their number, 15, to give a mean of 1.50 μmol/24 h. This familiar process is conveniently expressed by the following symbols:

$$\bar{x} = \frac{\sum x}{n}$$

$\bar{x}$ (pronounced "x bar") signifies the mean; x is each of the values of urinary lead; n is the number of these values; and Σ, the Greek capital sigma (English "S"), denotes "sum of". A major disadvantage

Statistics at Square One, XIth edition. By M.J. Campbell and T.D.V. Swinscow. Published 2009 by Blackwell Publishing, ISBN: 9781405191005.

of the mean is that it is sensitive to outlying points. For example, replacing 2.2 by 22 in Table 1.2 increases the mean to 2.82 μmol/24h, whereas the median will be unchanged.

A feature of the mean is that it is the value that minimizes the sum of the *squares* of the observations from a point, in contrast to the median which minimizes the sum of the absolute differences from a point (Chapter 1). For the data in Table 1.2, the first observation is 0.6 and the square of the difference from the mean is $(0.6 - 1.5)^2 = 0.81$. The sum of the squares for all the observations is 9.96 (see Table 2.1). No value other than 1.50 will give a smaller sum. It is also true that the sum of the differences (i.e. allowing both negative and positive values) of the observations from the mean will always be zero.

As well as measures of location we need measures of how variable the data are. We met two of these measures, the range and interquartile range, in Chapter 1.

The range is an important measurement, for figures at the top and bottom of it denote the findings furthest removed from the generality. However, they do not give much indication of the average spread of observations about the mean. This is where the standard deviation (SD) comes in.

The theoretical basis of the standard deviation is complex and need not trouble the user. We will discuss sampling and populations in Chapter 4. A practical point to note here is that, when the population from which the data arise have a distribution that is approximately "Normal" (or Gaussian), then the standard deviation provides a useful basis for interpreting the data in terms of probability.

The Normal distribution is represented by a family of curves defined uniquely by two parameters, which are the mean and the standard deviation of the population. The curves are always symmetrically bell shaped, but the extent to which the bell is compressed or flattened out depends on the standard deviation of the population. However, the mere fact that a curve is bell shaped does not mean that it represents a Normal distribution, because other distributions may have a similar sort of shape.

Many biological characteristics conform to a Normal distribution closely enough for it to be commonly used—for example, heights of adult men and women, blood pressures in a healthy population, random errors in many types of laboratory measurements, and biochemical data. Figure 2.1 shows a Normal curve calculated from

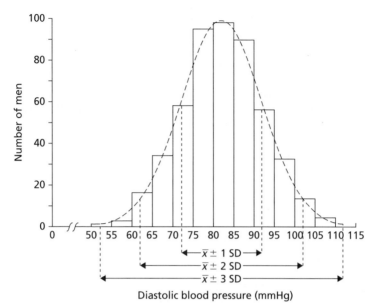

Figure 2.1 Normal curve calculated from diastolic blood pressures. 500 men, mean 82 mmHg, standard deviation 10 mmHg.

the diastolic blood pressures of 500 men, mean 82 mmHg, standard deviation 10 mmHg. The limits representing ±1 SD, ±2 SD, and ±3 SD about the mean are marked. A more extensive set of values is given in Table A (Appendix).

The reason why the standard deviation is such a useful measure of the scatter of the observations is this: if the observations follow a Normal distribution, a range covered by one standard deviation above the mean and one standard deviation below it ($\bar{x} \pm 1$ SD) includes about 68% of the observations; a range of two standard deviations above and two below ($\bar{x} \pm 22$ SD) about 95% of the observations; and of three standard deviations above and three below ($\bar{x} \pm 3$ SD) about 99.7% of the observations. Consequently, if we know the mean and standard deviation of a set of observations, we can obtain some useful information by simple arithmetic. By putting one, two, or three standard deviations above and below the mean, we can estimate the range of values that would be expected to include about 68%, 95%, and 99.7% of the observations.

Standard deviation from ungrouped data

The standard deviation is a summary measure of the differences of each observation from the mean of all the observations. If the differences themselves were added up, the positive would exactly balance the negative and so their sum would be zero. Consequently the squares of the differences are added. The sum of the squares is then divided by the number of observations *minus one* to give the mean of the squares, and the square root is taken to bring the measurements back to the units we started with. (The division by the number of observations *minus one* instead of the number of observations itself to obtain the mean square is because "degrees of freedom" must be used. In these circumstances they are one less than the total. The theoretical justification for this need not trouble the user in practice.) However, consider having only one observation in a data set. In this case the mean of the data is just that point. If we used a divisor of n, then we would have the variance = $0/1 = 0$. You might say, well that is true, the variance is zero, because there is no variability about that point. However we are trying to estimate the variance of the *population* (see Chapter 4). If we used $n - 1$ we get $0/0$ which is not estimable, which is also true when trying to estimate the variance of a group from a single observation.

To gain an intuitive feel for degrees of freedom, consider if we had a row of n fence posts. How many fence panels would we need to make a fence? The answer is $n - 1$. Once we know where the first fence post is, this determines where the others are. Thus, we need to estimate the mean before we can calculate the standard deviation and the mean determines where the data "are". The calculation of the standard deviation is illustrated in Table 2.1 with the 15 readings in the preliminary study of urinary lead concentrations (Table 1.2). The readings are set out in column (1). In column (2) the difference between each reading and the mean is recorded. The sum of the differences is 0. In column (3) the differences are squared, and the sum of those squares is given at the bottom of the column.

The sum of the squares of the differences (or deviations) from the mean, 9.96, is now divided by the total number of observation minus one, to give a quantity known as the *variance*. Thus,

$$\text{Variance} = \frac{\sum(x - \bar{x})^2}{n - 1}.$$

Table 2.1 Calculation of standard deviation.

(1) Lead Concentration (μmol/24 h)	(2) Differences From mean $x - \bar{x}$	(3) Differences Squared $(x - \bar{x})^2$
0.1	−1.4	1.96
0.4	−1.1	1.21
0.6	−0.9	0.81
0.8	−0.7	0.49
1.1	−0.4	0.16
1.2	−0.3	0.09
1.3	−0.2	0.04
1.5	0	0
1.7	0.2	0.04
1.9	0.4	0.16
1.9	0.4	0.16
2.0	0.5	0.25
2.2	0.7	0.49
2.6	1.1	1.21
3.2	1.7	2.89
Total 22.5	0	9.96

$n = 15$, $\bar{x} = 1.50$.

In this case we find:

$$\text{Variance} = \frac{9.96}{14} = 0.7114 \ (\mu\text{mol}/24 \text{ h})^2.$$

Finally, the square root of the variance provides the standard deviation:

$$\text{SD} = \sqrt{\frac{\Sigma(x - \bar{x})^2}{n-1}}, \qquad (2.1)$$

from which we get:

$$\text{SD} = \sqrt{0.7114} = 0.843 \ \mu\text{mol}/24 \text{ h}.$$

This procedure illustrates the structure of the standard deviation, in particular that the two extreme values 0.1 and 3.2 contribute most to the sum of the differences squared.

Standard deviation from grouped data

We can also calculate a standard deviation for count variables. For example, in addition to studying the lead concentration in the urine of 140 children, the pediatrician asked how often each of them had been examined by a doctor during the year. After collecting the information, he tabulated the data shown in Table 2.2 columns (1) and (2). The mean is calculated by multiplying column (1) by column (2), adding the products, and dividing by the total number of observations. Thus the mean number of visits is 455/140 = 3.25.

As we did for continuous data, to calculate the standard deviation, we subtract the mean from each of the observations in turn and then square it. In this case the observation is the number of visits, but because we have several children in each class, shown in column (2), each squared number (column (4)) must be multiplied by the number of children. The sum of squares is given at the foot of column (5), namely 218.2500. We then use the formula to find the variance:

$$\text{Variance} = \frac{218.25}{139} = 1.57$$

and

$$\text{SD} = \sqrt{1.57} = 1.25.$$

Table 2.2 Calculation of the standard deviation from count data.

(1) Number of visits to or by doctor	(2) Number of children	(3) Col (1) − 3.25	(4) Col (3) squared	(5) Col (2) × Col (4)
0	2	−3.25	10.5625	21.1250
1	8	−2.25	5.0625	40.5000
2	27	−1.25	1.5625	42.1875
3	45	−0.25	0.0625	2.8125
4	38	0.75	0.5625	21.3750
5	15	1.75	3.0625	45.9375
6	4	2.75	7.5625	30.2500
7	1	3.75	14.0625	14.0625
Total	140			218.2500

The use of OpenStat to calculate these statistics is shown in Chapter 14.

Note that although the number of visits is not Normally distributed, the distribution is reasonably symmetrical about the mean. The approximate 95% range is given by:

$$3.25 - 2 \times 1.25 = 0.75 \text{ to } 3.25 + 2 \times 1.25 = 5.75$$

This excludes two children with no visits and five children with six or more visits. Thus there are 7 of 140 = 5.0% outside the theoretical 95% range.

It is common for discrete quantitative variables to have what is known as a *skewed* distribution, that is, they are not symmetrical.

Clues to lack of symmetry from derived statistics are:
- The mean and the median differ considerably.
- The standard deviation is of the same order of magnitude as the mean, but the observations must be non-negative.

Sometimes a transformation will convert a skewed distribution into a symmetrical one. When the data are counts, such as number of visits to a doctor, often the square root transformation will help, and if there are no zero or negative values a logarithmic transformation may render the distribution more symmetrical.

Data transformation

An anesthetist measures the pain of a procedure using a 100 mm visual analogue scale on seven patients. The results are given in Table 2.3, together with the $\log_e$ transformation (the **ln** button on a calculator).

The data are plotted in Figure 2.2, which shows that the outlier does not appear so extreme in the logged data. The mean and median are 10.29 and 3 respectively, for the original data, with a standard deviation of 20.22. Where the mean is bigger than the median, the distribution is positively skewed. For the logged data, the mean and median are 1.24 and 1.10, respectively, which are relatively close,

Table 2.3 Results from pain score on seven patients (mm).

Original scale:	1,	1,	2,	3,	3,	6,	56
$\log_e$ scale:	0,	0,	0.69,	1.10	1.10,	1.79,	4.03

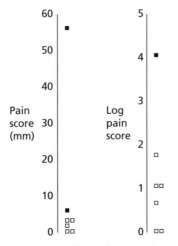

Figure 2.2 Dot plots of original and logged data from pain scores.

indicating that the logged data have a more symmetrical distribution. Thus it would be better to analyze the logged transformed data in statistical tests than using the original scale.

In reporting these results, the median of the raw data would be given, but it should be explained that the statistical test was carried out on the transformed data. Note that the median of the logged data is the same as the log of the median of the raw data—however, this is not true for the mean. The mean of the logged data is not necessarily equal to the log of the mean of the raw data. The anti-log (**exp** on a calculator) of the mean of the logged data is known as the *geometric* mean, and is often a better summary statistic than the mean, for data from positively skewed distributions. For these data the geometric mean is 3.45 mm.

Several points can be made:
- If two groups are to be compared, a transformation that reduces the skewness of an outcome variable often results in the stand-ard deviations of the variable in the two groups being similar.
- A log transform is the only one that will give sensible results on a back transformation.
- Transforming variables is not "cheating". Some variables are measured naturally on a log scale (e.g. pH).

Between subjects and within subjects standard deviation

If repeated measurements are made of, say, blood pressure on an individual, these measurements are likely to vary. This is within subject, or intrasubject, variability, and we can calculate a standard deviation of these observations. If the observations are close together in time, this standard deviation is often described as the *measurement error*. Measurements made on different subjects vary according to between subject, or intersubject, variability. If many observations were made on each individual, and the average taken, then we can assume that the intrasubject variability has been averaged out and the variation in the average values is due solely to the intersubject variability. Single observations on individuals clearly contain a mixture of intersubject and intrasubject variation, but we cannot separate the two since the within subject variability cannot be estimated with only one observation per subject. The *coefficient of variation* (CV%) is the intrasubject standard deviation divided by the mean, expressed as a percentage. It is often quoted as a measure of repeatability for biochemical assays, when an assay is carried out on several occasions on the same sample. It has the advantage of being independent of the units of measurement, but also it has numerous theoretical disadvantages. It is usually nonsensical to use the coefficient of variation as a measure of between subject variability.

The mode

The mode is the most common value and along with the mean and the median is a measure of location. It can be used for grouped continuous data, for count data and for categorical data. For example, in Table 1.4 the modal value of the distribution is 2.0–2.4 (µmol/24 hr) and in Table 2.2 the modal number of visits to a doctor is 3. The mode is only used for describing data.

Common questions

When should I quote the mean and when should I quote the median to describe my data?

It is a commonly held misapprehension that for Normally distributed data one uses the mean, and for non-Normally distributed data one uses the median. Alas, this is not so: if the data are approximately Normally distributed, the mean and the median will be close; if the data are not Normally distributed, then both the mean and the median may give useful information. Consider a variable that takes the value 1 for males and 0 for females. This is clearly not Normally distributed. However, the mean gives the proportion of males in the group, whereas the median merely tells us which group contained more than 50% of the people. Similarly, the mean from ordered categorical variables can be more useful than the median, if the ordered categories can be given meaningful scores. For example, a lecture might be rated as 1 (poor) to 5 (excellent). The usual statistic for summarizing the result would be the mean. For some outcome variables (such as cost), one might be interested in the mean, whatever the distribution of the data, since from the mean can be derived the total cost for a group. However, in the situation where there is a small group at one extreme of a distribution (e.g. annual income), the median will be more "representative" of the distribution.

When should I use a standard deviation to summarize variability?

The standard deviation is only interpretable as a summary measure for variables that have approximately symmetric distributions. It is often used to describe the characteristics of a group, for example, in the first table of a paper describing a clinical trial. It is often used, in my view incorrectly, to describe variability for measurements that are not plausibly normal, such as age. For these variables, the range or interquartile range is a better measure. The standard deviation should not be confused with the *standard error*, which is described in Chapter 4 and where the distinction between the two is spelled out.

Formula appreciation

We can see from formula (2.1) that values a long way from the mean contribute much more to the variance and standard deviation. This is confirmed in Table 2.1, which shows that the two extreme values contribute nearly half the value of the variance. Note that in Table 2.2, the groups contributing the most to the variance are not the most extreme ones, since the weighting is less for these groups.

Reading and displaying summary statistics

- In general, display means to one more significant digit than the original data, and standard deviations to two significant figures more. Try to avoid the temptation to spurious accuracy offered by computer printouts and calculator displays!
- Consider carefully if the quoted summary statistics correctly summarize the data. If a mean and standard deviation are quoted, is it reasonable to assume 95% of the population are within 2 SD of the mean? (Hint if the mean and standard deviation are about the same size, and if the observations must be positive, then the distribution will be skewed.)

Exercises

2.1 In the campaign against smallpox, a doctor inquired into the number of times 150 people aged 16 and over in an Ethiopian village had been vaccinated. He obtained the following figures: never, 12 people; once, 24; twice, 42; three times, 38; four times, 30; five times, 4. What is the mean number of times those people had been vaccinated and what is the standard deviation? Is the standard deviation a good measure of variation in this case?

2.2 Referring to the data in Exercise 1.1

    (a) Obtain the mean and standard deviation, and an approximate 95% range. Which points are excluded from the range mean -2 SD to mean $+ 2$ SD? What proportion of the data is excluded?

    (b) Playing with the data: see how changing the value 1.24 to 2.24 affects the statistics found in (a).

2.3 The following data were found in a study of asthmatic children. What are the best ways of graphically displaying the summaries of these data?

    (a) Peak flow: data quantitative and symmetrically distributed.

    (b) Number of episodes of wheeziness per day: data quantitative and with skewed distribution.

    (c) Social class of the child's parents: data qualitative and categorical.

CHAPTER 3

Summary statistics for binary data

Summarizing one binary variable

Recall that binary data only take one of two values such as "alive" or "dead", "male" or "female". We assign values 0 and 1 to the two states. For a single variable there are two ways of summarizing the information, proportions and odds. Proportions can be classified as risks or rates.

Consider 10 observations:

1 1 1 1 1 0 0 0 0 0

We could say that 5 out of 10 observations were 1, that is, a proportion 0.5 or a percentage 50% were 1. A proportion that is common in medicine is a *prevalence*. This is defined as the number of people in a population with a particular condition divided by the number of people in the population. This is sometimes multiplied by a round number such as 1000, so we have the prevalence per thousand, which is easier to understand. For example, the prevalence of type II diabetes is currently 0.003 or 3 per thousand people.

A proportion is a special sort of ratio, in that it must lie between 0 and 1. Another sort of ratio is a *rate*. This is the proportion of events that occur *within a given time period*. For example, the population of the UK is approximately 60 000 000. Every year about 600 000 people die. Thus the *crude mortality rate* for the UK is 600 000/60 000 000 = 1/100 or 0.01. This is often expressed per 1000, so that we say the crude mortality rate for the UK is about 10 per thousand *per year*. If the data referred to earlier arose because we followed up a group of 10 people for (say) a year and

Statistics at Square One, XIth edition. By M.J. Campbell and T.D.V. Swinscow.
Published 2009 by Blackwell Publishing, ISBN: 9781405191005.

5 developed a disease, then we often refer to the proportion as a *risk* of developing the disease. Strictly speaking, epidemiologists would call this an *incidence rate* and would require a time period to be specified. When one hears a risk quoted, always ask over what period of time. (After all, in the long run, the risk of death is one!)

An alternative way of looking at the 10 observations is to say that out of the 10 observations 5 observations were 1, and 5 were 0, that is, a ratio of 5:5, or what is known as an *odds* of 1 to 1. Statisticians drop the "to 1" as being understood. We might say something has a fifty-fifty chance, meaning a probability of 0.5. Odds are commonly used amongst the horse racing fraternity, where odds of 10 to 1 mean that out of 11 races they would expect a horse to win only once. Usually in betting, odds are bigger than one (since bookmakers would not quote you odds on something they thought is likely to happen). However, odds can be less than one, and so, unlike proportions, their only restriction is that they must be positive. In general, if you have x events and y non-events, the odds of an event are x/y and the proportion is $x/(x + y)$. It is a simple matter to relate odds (o) to proportions (p). The *odds* of an event are $o = p/(1 - p)$. Thus the odds are the ratio of the proportion of 1's to the proportion of 0's. Rewriting the equation, we find that $p = o/(1 + o)$. Thus an odds of 1 implies a proportion of 0.5.

Summarizing the relationship between two variables

Things become more interesting when we have two groups, and we will start with what is known as a 2×2 contingency table (it actually has three columns but the totals are not included in the description) as shown in Table 3.1.

We express the risk in group 1 as $p_1 = a/(a + b)$ and the risk in group 2 as $c/(c + d)$.

Table 3.1 2×2 Contingency table for comparison of two groups.

	Outcome		Total
	Positive	Negative	
Group 1	a	b	a + b
Group 2	c	d	c + d

Table 3.2 Results from the isoniazid trial after 6 months follow-up.[1]

	Dead	Alive	Total
Placebo	21	110	131
Isoniazid	11	121	132

As an example, consider Zar *et al.* who report on a trial of isoniazid for the treatment of tuberculosis in children with HIV.[1] The
outcome was death after 6 months follow-up. The results are given
in Table 3.2.

Under the placebo there was a risk of $p_1 = a/(a + b) = 21/131 =$
0.160 of dying 6 months after randomization. In the isoniazid
group, the risk was $p_2 = c/(c + d) = 11/132 = 0.083$.

To compare two proportions, what we really want is to look at
the *contrast* between differing therapies. We can do this by looking
at either the difference in risks or the ratio of risks.

Consider the difference in risk first. If we ignore the sign, this is
sometimes known as the *absolute risk difference (ARD)*, or if the risk
in the intervention group is lower than the control as the *absolute
risk reduction.*

Thus ARD $= |p_2 - p_1|$ (where the "||"means ignore the sign)

The difference in risks in this case is $0.160 - 0.083 = 0.077$ or
7.7%. One way of thinking about this is if 100 patients were
treated under placebo and 100 treated under isoniazid, we would
expect 16 to have died on placebo and 8.3 on isoniazid. Thus an
extra 7.7 died under placebo. Another way of looking at this is
to ask: how many patients would be treated for one extra person
to be saved by isoniazid? If 7.7 extra deaths resulted from treating 100 patients per group, and so $100/7.7 = 13$ patients per group
would be treated for 1 death to be saved in the intervention group.
Thus roughly if 13 patients were treated to placebo and 13 to isoniazid, we would expect 1 fewer patient to die on isoniazid. This
is known as the *number needed to treat* (NNT) (or if the treatment is
harmful, the number needed to treat for harm, NNTH) and is simply expressed as the inverse of the absolute risk difference.[2]

Thus NNT $= 1/|p_2 - p_1|$

The NNT has been suggested by Sackett *et al.*[3] as a useful and clinically intuitive way of thinking about the outcome of a clinical trial.

For example, in a clinical trial of pravastatin against usual therapy to prevent coronary events in men with moderate hypercholestremia and no history of myocardial infarction, the NNT is 42. Thus you would have to treat 42 men with prevastatin to prevent one extra coronary event, compared with the usual therapy. It is claimed that this is easier to understand than the relative risk reduction, or other summary statistics, and can be used to decide whether an effect is "large" by comparing the NNT for different therapies.

However, it is important to realize that comparison between NNTs can only be made if the baseline risks are similar. Thus, suppose a new therapy managed to reduce 5 year mortality of Creutzfeldt–Jakob disease from 100% on standard therapy to 90% on the new treatment. This would be a major breakthrough and has an NNT of $1/(1 - 0.9) = 10$. In contrast, a drug that reduced mortality from 50% to 40% would also have an NNT of 10, but would have much less impact.

We can also express the outcome from the isoniazid trial as a *risk ratio* or *relative risk (RR)*, which is the ratio of the two risks, experimental risk divided by control risk.

$$RR = p_2/p_1 = \frac{a(c + d)}{c(a + b)} \tag{3.1}$$

This is also sometimes called the *incidence rate ratio (IRR)*. In the isoniazid trial RR $= 0.083/0.16 = 0.52$.

With a relative risk less than one, we can also consider the relative risk reduction (RRR).

$$RRR = (p_1 - p_2)/p_1$$

This is easily shown to be $1 - RR$ and is often expressed as a percentage. Thus a child in the isoniazid trial has $1 - 0.52 = 0.48 = 48\%$ reduced risk of death in 6 months compared with placebo. In epidemiology, we can regard the isoniazid group as "exposed" and the placebo group as "unexposed". The RRR is then known as the prevented fraction in the exposed. In Chapter 14, Table 3.2 is analyzed using *OpenEpi*, which produces not only the estimates discussed in this chapter but also measures of uncertainty (confidence intervals) which are to be discussed in Chapter 5.

We can also summarize the trial in terms of odds. The odds of death on the placebo are $(21/131)/(110/131) = 21/110 = 0.191$ and on isoniazid they are $11/121 = 0.091$.

Table 3.3 Odds ratios and relative risks for different values of absolute risks.

p_2	p_1	Relative risk p_2/p_1	Odds ratio $\dfrac{p_2/(1-p_2)}{p_1/(1-p_1)}$
0.1	0.05	2.00	2.11
0.3	0.15	2.00	2.42
0.5	0.25	2.00	3.00
0.7	0.35	2.00	4.33

$$\text{The odds ratio (OR)} = \frac{p_2/(1-p_2)}{p_1/(1-p_1)}$$

In the notation of Table 3.1, this can be shown to be:

$$\text{OR} = \frac{ad}{bc} \tag{3.2}$$

In this case the OR $= 0.091/0.191 = 0.48$. In this case the odds ratio has almost the same value as the relative risk.

The odds ratio and the relative risk are related by:

$$\text{OR} = \frac{\text{RR}(1-p_1)}{(1-p_1\text{RR})} \tag{3.3}$$

We illustrate this relationship in Table 3.3. This demonstrates an important fact: the odds ratio is a close approximation to the relative risk when the baseline risk is low, but is a poor approximation if the baseline risk is high.

Treatments can do harm as well as good. As an example, consider Kennedy *et al.* who report on the study of acetazolamide and furosemide versus standard therapy for the treatment of post-hemorrhagic ventricular dilatation (PHVD) in premature babies.[4] The outcome was death or a shunt placement by 1 year of age. The results are given in Table 3.4.

Here the risk in the control group is 0.46 and in the intervention group it is 0.65. The relative risk of death or shunt in the intervention group compared with standard therapy is 1.42. This can be

Table 3.4 Results from the PHVD trial.[4]

	Death/shunt	No death/shunt	Total
Standard therapy	35	41	76
Drug plus standard therapy	49	26	75

expressed as a 42% increased risk (not an increase of 142% as is sometimes suggested). The NNTH is $1/|0.46 - 0.65| = 5.3 \sim 6$, so only 6 children need to be treated in each group for one extra to experience harm.

As a ratio of two numbers, the relative risk hides the actual size of the numbers. Thus a relative risk of 2 could be 8 people out of 10 having an event compared with 4 people out of 10, or it could be 2 people out of 1000 having an event compared with 1 person out of 1000. These have a completely different interpretation. This when a relative risk is quoted *always* ask about the absolute risks as well, so that a proper interpretation can be made.

For example, the risk of deep vein thrombosis in women on a new type of contraceptive is 30 per 100 000 women years, compared to 15 per 100 000 women years on the standard type. Thus the relative risk is 2, which shows that the new type of contraceptive carries quite a high risk of deep vein thrombosis. However, an individual woman need not be unduly concerned since she has a probability of 0.0003 of getting a deep vein thrombosis in 1 year on the new drug, which is much less than if she were pregnant!

Relative risks versus odds ratios

The odds ratio may not seem like an intuitively obvious statistic, but it has some useful properties. Consider an exposure which in low risk group has been found to double one's risk of disease. What would happen in a high risk population, where say the risk of the disease in the unexposed group was already over 50%? Clearly one cannot simply multiply the risk by the incidence in the unexposed to get the risk in the exposed, since one would get a risk greater than 1, (i.e. more than certain!). However, there are no such problems with the odds ratio.

A further use for the odds ratio arises when the data come from a cross-sectional study or a case–control study (see Chapter 14 for

Table 3.5 2×2 Table for association studies.

		Condition A		Total
		Present	Absent	
Condition B	Present	*a*	*b*	*a + b*
	Absent	*c*	*d*	*c + d*
	Total	*a + c*	*b + d*	

Table 3.6 Association between hay fever and eczema in 11 year old children.[5,6]

	Hay fever present	Hay fever absent	Total
Eczema present	141	420	561
Eczema absent	928	13525	14453
Total	1069	13945	15014

a discussion of these types of studies). In a case–control study, it is not possible to calculate a relative risk directly, but one can use the odds ratio to estimate the relative risk.

Suppose there are two conditions A and B, which are present or absent, and we wish to see if there is an association between the two. We rewrite Table 3.1 as Table 3.5.

We can argue across the rows:

Given condition B is present, the odds for A being present are *a/b*.

Given condition B is absent, the odds for A being present are *c/d*.

Thus the odds ratio for A being present, given B being present relative to B being absent is (a/b)/(c/d) = ad/bc. We say 'the odds ratio of A *given* B = ad/bc.

However we can also argue down the columns.

Given condition A is present, the odds for B being present are *a/c*.

Given condition A is absent, the odds for B being present are *b/d*.

Thus the odds ratio for B given A is (a/c)/(b/d) = ad/bc.

Thus the odds ratio for A given B is the same as the odds ratio for B given A.

To illustrate this consider Table 3.6, showing the prevalence of hay fever and eczema in a cross-sectional survey of 11 year old children.[5,6]

If a child has hay fever, the risk of eczema is 141/1069 = 0.132 and the odds are 141/928 = 0.152. If a child does not have hay fever, the risk of eczema is 420/13945 = 0.030 and the odds are

420/13525 = 0.031. Thus the relative risk of having eczema, given that a child has hay fever, is 0.132/0.030, which is 4.40. We can also find the odds ratio of having eczema given that a child has hay fever as 0.152/0.031 = 4.90.

We can consider the table the other way around, and ask what is the risk of hay fever given that a child has eczema. In this case, the two risks are 141/561 = 0.251 and 928/14453 = 0.064, and the relative risk is 0.251/0.064 = 3.92. Thus the relative risk of hay fever given that a child has eczema is 3.92, which is not the same as the relative risk of eczema given that a child has hay fever, which is 4.40. However, the two respective odds are 141/420 = 0.336 and 928/13525 = 0.069, and the odds ratio is 0.336/0.069 = 4.87, which to the limits of rounding is the same as the odds ratio for eczema, given a child has hay fever of 4.90.

The fact that the two odds ratios are the same can be seen from the fact that

$$OR = \frac{141 \times 13525}{928 \times 420}$$

and this remains the same if we switch rows and columns.

Thus we can either say the children with hay fever have five times the odds of getting eczema, or that children with eczema have five times the odds of getting hay fever. This will be approximately true for risks because hay fever and eczema are quite rare in the population, but would not be true if the incidence was higher.

Another useful property of the odds ratio is that the odds ratio for an event *not* happening is just the inverse of the odds ratio for it happening. Thus, the odds ratio for *not* having eczema, given that a child has hay fever, is just 1/4.90 = 0.204. This is not true of the relative risk, where the relative risk for not getting eczema given a child has hay fever is (420/561)/(13525/14453) = 0.80, which is not 1/3.92 = 0.2551.

Odds ratios and case–control studies

The design of case–control and cohort studies will be discussed in Chapter 13. These relate exposure to some hazard to outcome in the form of disease or death. A cohort study measures exposure and then observes events to answer the question, *if* one is exposed to a hazard (E) what is the probability of disease D (i.e. Prob($D|E$))?

(This reads as the probability of disease *given* exposure. A case–control study argues the other way around. It measures events and looks backwards for exposure (i.e. Prob($E|D$)).

The outcome from a case–control study can be expressed as a 2×2 table as shown in Table 3.7.

Notice that the "outcome" in Table 3.1 has been replaced by whether a subject is a case or a control. Thus a "case" may be someone who has died and a "control" someone who is still alive. The odds ratio of being a case given exposure is ad/bc. It is tempting to think of the relative risk as $(a/(a + b))/(c/(c + d))$. However, we will demonstrate that this cannot be the case. Firstly, observe that we cannot think of $(a + c)/n$ as the prevalence of the disease, since in case–control studies the relative number of cases to controls can be decided by the investigator. It is common to use the same number of cases and controls, and yet one would not think that the prevalence was 50%. Similarly, the usual measure of the relative risk no longer holds.

Suppose the investigator decided to double the number of controls as shown in Table 3.8. It is a simple matter to show that the estimate of the "relative risk" is changed from $\{a/(a + b)\}/\{c/(c + d)\}$ to $\{a/(a + 2b)\}/\{c/(c + 2d)\}$, which are different when b and d are non-zero. However, the estimate of the odds ratio remains as ad/bc. Thus the odds ratio is unaffected by the case/control ratio, but the "relative risk" is. Since the risk of disease if someone is exposed to

Table 3.7 2×2 Table for a case–control study.

	Case	Control	Total
Exposed	*a*	*b*	*a + b*
Not exposed	*c*	*d*	*c + d*
Total	*a + c*	*b + d*	*n*

Table 3.8 2×2 Table for a case–control study with double the number of controls.

	Case	Control	Total
Exposed	*a*	2*b*	*a + b*
Not exposed	*c*	2*d*	*c + d*
Total	*a + c*	2*b + 2d*	

a hazard cannot be related to how many controls the investigator chose, one can see that the estimator of the relative risk in a case–control study is invalid.

However, when the assumption of a low absolute risk holds true (which is usually the situation for case–control studies), then the odds ratio and the relative risk are close, and so in this case the odds ratio is assumed to approximate the relative risk that would have been obtained if a cohort study had been conducted instead of a case–control study.

Paired alternatives

Sometimes it is possible to record the results of treatment or some sort of test or investigation as one of two alternatives. For instance, two treatments or tests might be carried out on pairs obtained by matching individuals, or the pairs might consist of successive treatments of the same individual. The result might then be recorded as "responded or did not respond", "improved or did not improve", "positive or negative", and so on. These types of studies may be crossover trials or matched case–control studies and are described in Chapter 13. The results can be set out as shown in Table 3.9.

The proportion of those who responded on treatment A is $p_A = (e + f)/n$

The proportion which responded on treatment B is $p_B = (e + g)/n$

The difference in the proportions of responses is $p_A - p_B = (f - g)/n$

Note that we do not need to know the separate values of the number of pairs who both responded or both did not respond to calculate this difference.

Table 3.9 can be rewritten as a 2×2 table as shown in Table 3.10, but now the numbers in the table refer to the number of *pairs*.

It can be shown that the odds of responding to A compared to B are:

$$OR_{paired} = f/g$$

Note that here we do not need to know e, h, or n. This seems rather counterintuitive. However, consider a situation where we want to know whether one of two drugs is better. We use a crossover design in which each patient gets both drugs in random order. Then if the patient responds to both, this does not tell us which of the two is better. Similarly if the patient does not respond to either,

Table 3.9 Results from a matched or paired study.

Member of pair receiving treatment A	Member of pair receiving treatment B	Pairs of patients
Responded	Responded	e
Responded	Did not respond	f
Did not respond	Responded	g
Did not respond	Did not respond	h
Total		n

Table 3.10 Layout for paired data.

		Subject Getting B		
		Positive	Negative	Total
Subject	Positive	e	f	e + f
Getting A	Negative	g	h	g + h
Total		e + g	f + h	n

we have no information as to which is better. It is only when a patient responds to one and not the other do we glean any information as to which drug is better.

For example, a registrar in the gastroenterological unit of a large hospital in an industrial city sees a considerable number of patients with severe recurrent aphthous ulcer of the mouth. Claims have been made that a recently introduced preparation stops the pain of these ulcers and promotes quicker healing than existing preparations.

Over a period of 6 months, the registrar selected every patient with this disorder and paired them off, as far as possible, by reference to age, sex, and frequency of ulceration. Finally she had 108 patients in 54 pairs. To one member of each pair, chosen by the toss of a coin, she gave treatment A, which she and her colleagues in the unit had hitherto regarded as the best; to the other member she gave the new treatment, B. Both forms of treatment are local applications, and they cannot be made to look alike. Consequently, to avoid bias in the assessment of the results, a colleague recorded the results of treatment without knowing which patient in each pair had which treatment. The results are shown in Table 3.11.

The observed difference in proportions is:

$$23/54 - 10/54 = 0.241$$

Table 3.11 Data aphthous ulcer study.

		Treatment B	
		Responded	Did not respond
Treatment A	Responded	16	10
	Did not respond	23	5

Table 3.12 Methods of summarizing a binary outcome in a two group prospective* study: Risk in group 1 (control) is p_1, risk in group 2 is p_2.

Term	Formula	Observed in the isoniazid trial
Absolute risk difference (ARD)	$\lvert p_1 - p_2 \rvert$	$0.160 - 0.083 = 0.077$
Relative risk (RR)	p_2/p_1	$0.083/0.160 = 0.52$
Relative risk reduction (RRR)	$(p_1 - p_2)/p_1$	$(0.160 - 0.083/0.16 = 0.48$
Number needed to treat or harm (NNT or NNTH))	$1/\lvert p_1 - p_2 \rvert$	$1/0.077 \approx 13$
Odds ratio (OR)	$\{p_2/(1 - p_2)\}/\{p_1/(1 - p_1)\}$	$(0.083/0.917)/(0.160/0.840) = 0.48$

*For example, a trial or a cohort study—not a case–control study.

The odds ratio is $10/23 = 0.43$. Thus the odds of responding on A are 0.43 times that of responding on B. We will explore these data further in Chapter 8 where paired data are tested using a McNemar's test.

Summary: choice of summary statistics for binary data from a non-matched study

Table 3.12 gives a summary of the different methods of summarizing a binary outcome for a prospective study such as a clinical trial.

Common questions

When should I quote an odds ratio and when should I quote a relative risk?

The odds ratio is difficult to understand and most people think of it as a relative risk anyway. Thus for prospective studies, the relative risk should be easy to derive and should be quoted, and not the odds ratio. For case–control studies, one has no option but to quote the odds ratio. For cross-sectional studies, one has a choice, and if it is not clear which variables are causal and which are outcome, then the odds ratio has the advantage of being symmetric, in that it gives the same answer if the causal and outcome variables are swapped. A major reason for quoting odds ratios is that they are the output from *logistic regression*, an advanced technique discussed in *Statistics at Square Two*.[7] These are quoted, even for prospective studies, because of the nice statistical properties of odds ratios. In this situation, it is important to label the odds ratios correctly, and consider situations in which they may not be good approximations to relative risks.

Formula appreciation

Equation (3.1) can be derived simply from Table 3.1, since the odds of a positive outcome in group 1 are a/b and those in group 2 are c/d so the ratio is ad/bc. In equation (3.3) one can see that if the RR is close to 1 it will also be close to the OR.

Reading and displaying summary statistics

- If a relative risk is quoted, is it in fact an odds ratio? Is it reasonable to assume that the odds ratio is a good approximation to a relative risk?
- *Always* ascertain the absolute risk difference, when considering relative risks.
- If an NNT is quoted, what are the absolute levels of risk? If you are trying to evaluate a therapy, does the absolute level of risk given in the paper correspond to what you might expect in your own patients?
- Always display measures of uncertainty about estimates (see Chapter 5).

Exercises

3.1 A recent advert in the medical press for clopidogrel reads as follows: "It's great to be a statistic! 20% relative risk reduction". A 20% relative risk reduction means that when patients given active treatment are compared with patients given placebo:
(a) 20% of those given the active treatment will benefit.
(b) We can be 20% sure that the treatment works.

(c) The difference in risks is 0.2.

(d) Risk in the treatment group is 80% of that in the control group.

3.2 The CURE study examined the use of clopidogrel and aspirin in acute coronary syndromes. It showed that the combined risk of cardiovascular death, stroke, and myocardial infarction was 11.4% in the placebo group and 9.3% in the clopidogrel group. The risk of major bleeding increased by 1% using clopidogrel and aspirin drugs.

(a) This can be described as a risk difference of 2.1%.

(b) This means the number needed to treat for one to benefit (NNTB) is around five.

(c) The data can be reported as a relative risk reduction of around 80%.

3.3 A report of the CURE study in the medical press read as follows: "Treating unstable angina and non-Q wave myocardial infarction with clopidogrel and aspirin resulted in a 20% reduction in the risk of myocardial infarction, stroke, and vascular death. The risk of major bleeding increased by 1% using clopidogrel and aspirin drugs".

(a) The report suggests that the benefit of treatment is much greater than the risk of bleeding.

(b) If both differences were reported as absolute risk differences, the reduction in vascular events would be 2.1% and the increased risk of bleeding would be 1.0%.

3.4 A pharmaceutical representative provides the following information on a randomized controlled trial of "Supersporin", a new antifungal treatment for fungal nail infection compared with oral terbinafine.

Number of patients

	"Supersporin" treated group	Terbinafine treated group
Cured at 12 weeks	40	20
Not cured > 12 weeks	60	80

Which ONE of the following values is the ABSOLUTE REDUCTION in the risk of being cured in the "Supersporin" group? Select ONE option only.

20%, 40%, 50%, 60%, 100%

3.5 How many patients would need to be treated with "Supersporin" to cure one patient with a fungal nail infection who would not have been cured with terbinafine? Select ONE option only.

1, 2, 2.5, 5, 10

3.6 In a prospective study of 241 men and 222 women undergoing elective inpatient surgery, 37 men and 61 women suffered nausea and vomiting in the recovery room.[8] Find the relative risk and odds ratio for nausea and vomiting for women compared to men.

References

1. Zar HJ, Cotton MF, Strauss S, *et al*. Effect of isoniazid prophylaxi on mortality and incidence of tuberculosis in children with HIV: randomised controlled trial. *BMJ* 2007;**334**:136–9.
2. Cook RJ and Sackett DL. The number needed to treat: a clinically useful measure of treatment effect. *BMJ* 1995;**310**:452–4.
3. Sackett DL, Richardson WS, Rosenberg W and Hayne RB. *Evidence-Based Medicine: How to Practice and Teach EBM*. New York: Churchill Livingstone, 1997.
4. International PHVD Drug Trial Group. International randomised controlled trial of acetazolamide and furosemide in post-haemorrhagic ventricular dilatation in infancy. *Lancet* 1998;**352**:433–40.
5. Strachan DP, Butland BK and Anderson HR. Incidence and prognosis of asthma and wheezing from early childhood to age 33 in a national British cohort. *BMJ* 1996;**312**:1195–9.
6. Bland JM and Altman DG. Statistics notes: the odds ratio. *BMJ* 2000;**320**:1468.
7. Campbell MJ. *Statistics at Square Two*, 2nd ed. Oxford: Wiley-Blackwell, 2006.
8. Myles PS, Mcleod ADM, Hunt JO and Fletcher H. Sex differences in speed of emergency and quality of recovery after anaesthetic: cohort study. *BMJ* 2001;**322**:710–11.

CHAPTER 4
Populations and samples

Populations

In statistics the term "population" has a slightly different meaning
from the one given to it in ordinary speech. It need not refer only
to people or to animate creatures—the population of Britain, for
instance, or the dog population of London. Statisticians also speak
of a population of objects, or events, or procedures, or observations, including things such as the quantity of lead in urine, visits
to the doctor, or surgical operations. A population is thus an aggre-
gate of creatures, things, cases, and so on.

Although a statistician should clearly define the relevant population, he or she may not be able to enumerate it exactly. For
instance, in ordinary usage, the population of England denotes the
number of people within England's boundaries, perhaps as enu-
merated at a census. But a physician might embark on a study to
try to answer the question "What is the average systolic blood pressure of Englishmen aged 40–59?" But who are the "Englishmen"
referred to here? Not all Englishmen live in England, and the social
and genetic background of those that do may vary. A surgeon may
study the effects of two alternative operations for gastric ulcer. But
how old are the patients? What sex are they? How severe is their
disease? Where do they live? And so on. The reader needs precise information on such matters to draw valid inferences from
the sample that was studied to the population being considered.
Statistics such as averages and standard deviations, when taken
from populations, are referred to as *population parameters*. They are
often denoted by Greek letters; the population mean is denoted

Statistics at Square One, XIth edition. By M.J. Campbell and T.D.V. Swinscow.
Published 2009 by Blackwell Publishing, ISBN: 9781405191005.

by μ (mu) and the standard deviation denoted by σ (lower case sigma).

Samples

A population commonly contains too many individuals to study conveniently, so an investigation is often restricted to one or more samples drawn from it. A well-chosen sample will contain most of the information about a particular population parameter, but the relation between the sample and the population must be such as to allow true inferences to be made about a population from that sample.

Consequently, the first important attribute of a sample is that every individual in the population from which it is drawn must have a known non-zero chance of being included in it; a natural suggestion is that these chances should be equal. We would like the choices to be made independently; in other words, the choice of one subject will not affect the chance of other subjects being chosen. To ensure this we make the choice by means of a process in which chance alone operates, such as spinning a coin or, more usually, the use of a table of random numbers. A limited table is given in the Table B (Appendix), and more extensive ones have been published.[1] A sample so chosen is called a random sample. The word "random" does not describe the sample as such, but the way in which it is selected.

To draw a satisfactory sample sometimes presents greater problems than to analyze statistically the observations made on it. A full discussion of the topic is beyond the scope of this book, and here we only offer an introduction.

Before drawing a sample, the investigator should define the population from which it is to come. Sometimes, he or she can completely enumerate its members before beginning analysis—for example, all the livers studied at necropsy over the previous year, all the patients aged 20–44 admitted to hospital with perforated peptic ulcer in the previous 20 months. In retrospective studies of this kind, numbers can be allotted serially from any point in the table to each patient or specimen. Suppose we have a population of size 150, and we wish to take a sample of size five. Table B contains a set of computer generated random digits arranged in groups of five. Choose any row or column, say the last column of five digits. Read only the first three digits, and go down the column starting with the first row. Thus we have 265, 881, 722, etc. If a number appears between 001 and 150 then we include it in our sample. Thus, in order, in the sample will be subjects numbered 24, 59, 107, 73, and 65. If necessary we can carry on down the next column to the left until the full sample is chosen.

The use of random numbers in this way is generally preferable to taking every alternate patient or every fifth specimen, or acting on some other such regular plan. The regularity of the plan can occasionally coincide by chance with some unforeseen regularity in the presentation of the material for study—for example, by hospital appointments being made from patients from certain practices on certain days of the week, or specimens being prepared in batches in accordance with some schedule.

As susceptibility to disease generally varies in relation to age, sex, occupation, family history, exposure to risk, inoculation state, country lived in or visited, and many other genetic or environmental factors, it is advisable to examine samples when drawn to see whether they are, on average, comparable in these respects. The random process of selection is intended to make them so, but sometimes it can by chance lead to disparities. To guard against this possibility the sampling may be stratified. This means that a framework is laid down initially, and the patients or objects of the study in a random sample are then allotted to the compartments of the framework. For instance, the framework might have a primary division into males and females and then a secondary division of each of those categories into five age groups, the result being a framework with 10 compartments. It is then important to bear in mind that the distributions of the categories on two samples made up on such a framework may be truly comparable, but they will not reflect the distribution of these categories in the population from which the sample is drawn unless the compartments in the framework have been designed with that in mind. For instance, equal numbers might be admitted to the male and female categories, but males and females are not equally numerous in the general population, and their relative proportions vary with age. This is known as stratified random sampling. For taking a sample from a long list, a compromise between strict theory and practicalities is known as a *systematic random sample*. In this case, we choose subjects a fixed interval apart on the list, say every tenth subject, but we choose the starting point within the first interval at random.

Unbiasedness and precision

The terms unbiased and precision have acquired special meanings in statistics. When we say that a measurement is *unbiased*, we mean that the average of a large set of unbiased measurements will be close to the true value. When we say it is *precise*, we mean that repeated measurements will be close to one another. However these may not necessarily be close to the true value. We would like a measurement that is both unbiased and precise. Some authors equate unbiasedness with accuracy, but this is not universal and others use the term accuracy to mean a measurement that is both unbiased and precise. Strike[2] gives a good discussion of the problem.

An estimate of a parameter taken from a random sample is known to be unbiased. As the sample size increases, it gets more precise.

Randomization

Another use of random number tables is to randomize the allocation of treatments to patients in a clinical trial. This ensures that there is no bias in treatment allocation and, in the long run, the subjects in each treatment group are comparable in both known and unknown prognostic factors. A common method is to use *blocked randomization*. This is to ensure that at regular intervals there are equal numbers in the two groups. Usual sizes for blocks are two, four, six, eight, and ten. Suppose we chose a block size of ten. A simple method using the table of random numbers given in Table B in the Appendix is to choose the first five unique digits in any row. If we chose the first row, the first five unique digits are 3, 5, 6, 8, and 4. Thus we would allocate the third, fourth, fifth, sixth, and eighth subjects to one treatment and the first, second, seventh, ninth, and tenth to the other. If the block size was less than ten, we would ignore digits bigger than the block size. To allocate further subjects to treatment, we carry on along the same row, choosing the next five unique digits for the first treatment. In randomized controlled trials, it is advisable to change the block size from time to time to make it more difficult to guess what the next treatment is going to be.

It is important to realize that patients in a randomized trial are *not* a random sample from the population of people with the disease in question but rather a highly selected set of eligible and willing patients. However, randomization ensures that in the long run, any differences in outcome in the two treatment groups are due solely to differences in treatment.

Variation between samples

Even if we ensure that every member of a population has a known, and usually an equal, chance of being included in a sample, it does not follow that a series of samples drawn from one population and fulfilling this criterion will be identical. They will show chance variations from one to another, and the variation may be slight or considerable. For example, a series of samples of the body temperature of healthy people would show very little variation from one to another, but the variation between samples of the systolic blood pressure would be considerable. Thus the variation between samples depends partly on the amount of variation in the population from which they are drawn.

Furthermore, it is a matter of common observation that a small sample is a much less certain guide to the population from which it was drawn than a large sample. In other words, the more members of a population that are included in a sample the more chance will that sample have of accurately representing the population, provided a random process is used to construct the sample. A consequence of this is that, if two or more samples are drawn from a population, the larger they are the more likely they are to resemble each other—again provided that the random technique is followed. Thus the variation between samples depends partly also on the size of the sample. Usually, however, we are not in a position to take a random sample; our sample is simply those subjects available for study. This is a "convenience" sample. For valid generalizations to be made, we would like to assert that our sample is in some way representative of the population as a whole, and for this reason the first stage in a report is to describe the sample, say by age, sex, and disease status, so that other readers can decide if it is representative of the type of patients they encounter.

Standard error of the mean

If we draw a series of samples and calculate the mean of the observations in each, we have a series of means. These means generally conform to a Normal distribution, and they often do so even if the observations from which they were obtained do not (see Exercise 4.3). This can be proven mathematically and is known as the "central limit theorem". The series of means, like the series of observations in each sample, has a standard deviation. The standard error of the mean of one sample is an estimate of the standard deviation that would be obtained from the means of a large number of samples drawn from that population.

As noted above, if random samples are drawn from a population, their means will vary from one to another. The variation depends on the variation of the population and the size of the sample. We do not know the variation in the population, so we use the variation in the sample as an estimate of it. This is expressed in the standard deviation. If we now divide the standard deviation by the square root of the number of observations in the sample, we have an estimate of the standard error of the mean, $SEM = SD/\sqrt{n}$. It is important to realize that we do not have to take repeated samples in order to estimate the standard error; there is sufficient information within a single sample. However, the concept is that, if we were to take repeated random samples from the population, this is how we would expect the mean to vary, purely by chance.

A general practitioner in Yorkshire has a practice which includes part of a town with a large printing works and some of the adjacent sheep farming country. With her patients' informed consent, she has been investigating whether the diastolic blood pressure of men aged 20–44 differs between the printers and the farmworkers. For this purpose, she has obtained a random sample of 72 printers and 48 farmworkers and calculated the mean and standard deviations, as shown in Table 4.1.

To calculate the standard errors of the two mean blood pressures, the standard deviation of each sample is divided by the square root of the number of the observations in the sample.

$$\text{Printers: } SEM = 4.5/\sqrt{72} = 0.53 \text{ mmHg}$$

$$\text{Farmers: } SEM = 4.2/\sqrt{48} = 0.61 \text{ mmHg}$$

Table 4.1 Mean diastolic blood pressures of printers and farmers.

	Number	Mean diastolic blood pressure (mmHg)	Standard deviation (mmHg)
Printers	72	88	4.5
Farmers	48	79	4.2

These standard errors may be used to study the significance of the difference between the two means, as described in successive chapters.

Standard error of a proportion or a percentage

Just as we can calculate a standard error associated with a mean, so we can also calculate a standard error associated with a percentage or a proportion. Here the size of the sample will affect the size of the standard error, but the amount of variation is determined by the value of the percentage or proportion in the population itself, and so we do not need an estimate of the standard deviation. For example, a senior surgical registrar in a large hospital is investigating acute appendicitis in people aged 65 and over. As a preliminary study, he examines the hospital case notes over the previous 10 years and finds that of 120 patients in this age group with a diagnosis confirmed at operation 73 (60.8%) were women and 47 (39.2%) were men.

If p represents one percentage, $100 - p$ represents the other. Then the standard error of each of these percentages is obtained by (1) multiplying them together, (2) dividing the product by the number in the sample, and (3) taking the square root:

$$\text{SE percentage} = \sqrt{\frac{p(100 - p)}{n}}$$

which for the appendicitis data given above is as follows:

$$\text{SE percentage} = \sqrt{\frac{60.8 \times 39.2}{120}} = 4.46$$

Problems with non-random samples

In general, we do not have the luxury of a random sample; we have to make do with what is available, a *convenience sample*. In order to be able to make generalizations, we should investigate whether biases could have crept in, which mean that the patients available are not typical. Common biases are:

- hospital patients are not the same as ones seen in the community;
- volunteers are not typical of non-volunteers;
- patients who return questionnaires are different from those who do not.

In order to persuade the reader that the patients included are typical, it is important to give as much detail as possible at the beginning of a report of the selection process and some demographic data such as age, sex, social class, and response rate.

Common questions

What is an acceptable response rate from a survey?

If one were taking a sample to estimate some population parameter, then one would like as high a response rate as possible. It is convention to accept 65–70% as reasonable. Note, however, that valid inferences can be made on much smaller response rates, provided no biases in response occur. If one has data on the non-responders such as age or gender, it is useful to report it with the responders, to see if there are any obvious discrepancies.

Given measurements on a sample, what is the difference between a standard deviation and a standard error?

A standard deviation is a sample estimate of the population parameter σ; that is, it is an estimate of the variability of the observations. Since the population is unique, it has a unique standard deviation, which may be large or small depending on how variable the observations are. We would not expect the sample standard deviation to get smaller because the sample gets larger. However, a large sample would provide a more precise estimate of the population standard deviation σ than a small sample.

A standard error, on the other hand, is a measure of precision of an estimate of a population parameter. A standard error is always attached to a parameter, and one can have standard errors of any estimate, such as mean, median, fifth centile, even the standard error of the standard deviation. Since one would expect the precision of the estimate to increase with the sample size, the standard error of an estimate will decrease as the sample size increases.

When should I use a standard deviation to describe data and when should I use a standard error?

It is a common mistake to try and use the standard error to describe data. Usually it is done because the standard error is smaller, and so the study appears more precise. Statistical software often gives both in a single command, with no guidance as to which to use.

If the purpose is to describe the data (e.g. so that one can see if the patients are typical) and if the data are plausibly Normal, then one should use the standard deviation (mnemonic D for Description and D for Deviation). These are the sort of result one would see in the first table of a paper. If the purpose is to describe the outcome of a study, for example, to estimate the prevalence of a disease, or the difference between two treatment groups, then one should use a standard error (or, better, a confidence interval; see Chapter 5) (mnemonic E for Estimate and E for Error). Thus, in a paper, one would *describe* the sample in the first table (and so give, say, SD of blood pressure, and age range) and give *estimates* of the effects in the second table (and so give SEs of blood pressure differences).

Reading and reporting populations and samples

- Report carefully how the sample was chosen. Were the subjects simply patients who happened to be about? Were they consecutive patients who satisfied certain criteria?
- Report differences in defining demographic factors between the sample and the remaining population.
- List the reasons for exclusions, and compare responders and non-responders for key variables. In questionnaire surveys, describe how target population was obtained, and give numbers of people who refused to complete the questionnaire or who were "not available".
- When reading a paper, from the information given ask whether the results are generalizable.

Exercises

4.1 The mean urinary lead concentration in 140 children was 2.18 μmol/24 h with standard deviation 0.87. What is the standard error of the mean?

4.2 In Table B (Appendix) giving random numbers between 0 and 9, what would one expect the distribution of the digits to look like. Without doing any involved calculation, estimate the mean.

4.3 For the first column of five digits in Table B, take the mean value of the five digits and do this for the first 20 rows of five digits in the column. Plot a histogram of these means and find their mean and standard deviation.

What would you expect a histogram of the means to look like?

What would you expect the mean of the 20 numbers to be? Given that the standard deviation of the numbers in Table B is 2.87, what do we expect the standard deviation of the means going to be? How does this compare to the observed standard error?

References

1. Machin D, Campbell MJ, Tan SB and Tan SZ. *Statistical Tables for the Design of Clinical Studies*, 3rd ed. Oxford: Wiley-Blackwell, 2009.
2. Strike PW. *Measurement and Control. Statistical Methods in Laboratory Medicine*. Oxford: Butterworth-Heinemann, 1991:255.

CHAPTER 5
Statements of probability and confidence intervals

We have seen that when a set of observations have a Normal distribution, multiples of the standard deviation mark certain limits on the scatter of the observations. For instance, 1.96 (or approximately 2) standard deviations above and 1.96 standard deviations below the mean (± 1.96 SD) mark the points within which 95% of the observations lie.

Reference ranges

We noted in Chapter 1 that 140 children had a mean urinary lead concentration of 2.18 μmol/24 h, with standard deviation 0.87. We assume that urinary lead concentrations are Normally distributed. In this case, the points that include 95% of the observations are $2.18 \pm (1.96 \times 0.87)$, giving an interval of 0.48 to 3.89. One of the children had a urinary lead concentration of just over 4.0 μmol/24 h. This observation is greater than 3.89 and so falls in the 5% beyond the 95% probability limits. We can say that the probability of each of such observations occurring is 5%. Another way of looking at this is to see that if one chose one child at random out of the 140, the chance that their urinary lead concentration exceeded 3.89, or was less than 0.48, is 5%. This probability is usually expressed as a fraction of 1 rather than of 100, and written $P < 0.05$.

Standard deviations thus set limits about which probability statements can be made. Some of these are set out in Table A (Appendix). To use Table A to estimate the probability of finding an observed value, say a urinary lead concentration of 4.8 μmol/24 h, in sampling from the same population of observations as the

Statistics at Square One, XIth edition. By M.J. Campbell and T.D.V. Swinscow. Published 2009 by Blackwell Publishing, ISBN: 9781405191005.

140 children provided, we proceed as follows. The distance of the new observation from the mean is $4.8 - 2.18 = 2.62$. How many standard deviations does this represent? Dividing the difference by the standard deviation gives $2.62/0.87 = 3.01$. This number is greater than 2.576 but less than 3.291 in Table A, so the probability of finding a deviation as large or more extreme than this lies between 0.01 and 0.001, which may be expressed as $0.001 < P < 0.01$. In fact Table A shows that the probability is very close to 0.0027. This probability is small, so the observation probably did not come from the same population as the 140 other children.

To take another example, the mean diastolic blood pressure of printers was found to be 88 mmHg and the standard deviation 4.5 mmHg. One of the printers had a diastolic blood pressure of 100 mmHg. The mean plus or minus 1.96 times its standard deviation gives the following two figures:

$$88 + (1.96 \times 4.5) = 96.8 \, \text{mmHg}$$

$$88 - (1.96 \times 4.5) = 79.2 \, \text{mmHg}$$

We can say therefore that only 1 in 20 (or 5%) of printers in the population from which the sample is drawn would be expected to have a diastolic blood pressure below 79 or above about 97 mmHg. These are the 95% limits. The 99.73% limits lie 3 SD below and three above the mean. The blood pressure of 100 mmHg noted in one printer thus lies beyond the 95% limit of 97 but within the 99.73% limit of 101.5 $(= 88 + (3 \times 4.5))$.

The 95% limits are often referred to as a "reference range". For many biological variables, they define what is regarded as the normal (meaning standard or typical) range. Anything outside the range is regarded as abnormal. Given a sample of disease free subjects, an alternative method of defining a normal range would be simply to define points that exclude 2.5% of subjects at the top end and 2.5% of subjects at the lower end. This would give an *empirical normal range*. Thus in the 140 children we might choose to exclude the three highest and three lowest values. However, it is much more efficient to use the mean $\pm$ 2 SD, unless the data set is quite large (say >400).

Confidence intervals

The means and their standard errors can be treated in a similar fashion. If a series of samples are drawn and the mean of each calculated,

95% of the means would be expected to fall within the range of two standard errors above and two below the mean of these means. This common mean would be expected to lie very close to the mean of the population. So the standard error of a mean provides a statement of probability about the difference between the mean of the population and the mean of the sample.

In our sample of 72 printers, the standard error of the mean was 0.53 mmHg. The sample mean plus or minus 1.96 times its standard error gives the following two figures:

$$88 + (1.96 \times 0.53) = 89.04 \, \text{mmHg}$$

$$88 - (1.96 \times 0.53) = 86.96 \, \text{mmHg}$$

This is called the 95% *confidence interval*, and we can say that there is only a 5% chance that the range 86.96 to 89.04 mmHg excludes the mean of the population. If we take the mean plus or minus three times its standard error, the interval would be 86.41 to 89.59. This is the 99.73% confidence interval, and the chance of this interval excluding the population mean is 1 in 370. Confidence intervals provide the key to a useful device for arguing from a sample back to the population from which it came.

The standard error for the percentage of male patients with appendicitis, described in Chapter 4, was 4.46. This is also the standard error of the percentage of female patients with appendicitis, since the formula remains the same if p is replaced by $100 - p$. With this standard error, we can get 95% confidence intervals for the two percentages:

$$60.8 \pm (1.96 \times 4.46) = 52.1 \text{ and } 69.5$$

$$39.2 \pm (1.96 \times 4.46) = 30.5 \text{ and } 47.9$$

These confidence intervals exclude 50%. Can we conclude that males are more likely to get appendicitis? This is the subject of the rest of the book, namely *inference*.

With small samples—say under 30 observations—larger multiples of the standard error are needed to set confidence limits. This subject is discussed under the *t* distribution (Chapter 7).

There is much confusion over the interpretation of the probability attached to confidence intervals. To understand it, we have to resort to the concept of repeated sampling. Imagine taking repeated samples of the same size from the same population.

For each sample calculate a 95% confidence interval. Since the samples are different, so are the confidence intervals. We know that 95% of these intervals will include the population parameter. However, without any additional information, we cannot say which ones! Thus with only one sample, and no other information about the population parameter, we can say there is a 95% chance of including the parameter in our interval. Note that this does not mean that we would expect with 95% probability that the mean from another sample is in this interval. In this case, we are considering differences between two sample means, which is the subject of the next chapter.

Large sample standard error of difference between means

Consider now the mean of the second sample. If the sample comes from the same population, its mean will also have a 95% chance of lying within 1.96 standard errors of the population mean, but if we do not know the population mean, we have only the means of our samples to guide us. Therefore, if we want to know whether they are likely to have come from the same population, we ask whether they lie within a certain range, represented by their standard errors, of each other.

If SD_1 represents the standard deviation of sample 1 and SD_2 the standard deviation of sample 2, n_1 the number in sample 1 and n_2 the number in sample 2, a formula denoting the standard error of the difference between two means is:

$$SE \text{ (diff)} = \sqrt{\left(\frac{SD_1^2}{n_1} + \frac{SD_2^2}{n_2} \right)} \tag{5.1}$$

$$\text{or } SE \text{ (diff)} = \sqrt{SE_1^2 + SE_2^2}$$

Large sample confidence interval for the difference in two means

From the data in Table 4.1, the general practitioner wants to compare the mean of the printers' blood pressures with the mean of the farmers' blood pressures.

Analyzing these figures in accordance with the formula given above, we have:

$$\text{SE (diff)} = \sqrt{\left(\frac{4.5^2}{72} + \frac{4.2^2}{48}\right)} = 0.805 \text{ mmHg}$$

The difference between the means is $88 - 79 = 9$ mmHg. For large samples, we can calculate a 95% confidence interval for the difference in means as:

$$9 - (1.96 \times 0.805) \text{ to } 9 + (1.96 \times 0.805)$$

which is:

$$7.42 \text{ to } 10.58 \text{ mmHg}$$

For a small sample, we need to modify this procedure, as described in Chapter 7.

Standard error of difference between percentages or proportions

The surgical registrar who investigated appendicitis cases, referred to in Chapter 4, wonders whether the percentages of men and women in the sample differ from the percentages of all the other men and women aged 65, and over who were admitted to the surgical wards during the same period. After excluding his sample of appendicitis cases, so that they are not counted twice, he makes a rough estimate of the number of patients admitted in those 10 years and finds it to be about 12–13 000. He selects a systematic random sample of 640 patients, of whom 363 (56.7%) were women and 277 (43.3%) men.

The percentage of women in the appendicitis sample was 60.8% and differs from the percentage of women in the general surgical sample by $60.8 - 56.7 = 4.1$%. Is this difference of any significance? In other words, could this have arisen by chance?

There are two ways of calculating the standard error of the difference between two percentages: one is based on the null hypothesis that the two groups come from the same population; the other on the alternative hypothesis that they are different. For Normally distributed variables, these two are the same if the standard deviations are assumed to be the same, but in the binary case the standard deviations depend on the estimates of the proportions, and so if these are different so are the standard deviations. Usually, however, even in the binary case, both methods give almost the same result.

Confidence interval for a difference in proportions or percentages

The calculation of the standard error of a difference in proportions $p_1 - p_2$ follows the same logic as the calculation of the standard error of two means; sum the squares of the individual standard errors and then take the square root. It is based on the alternative hypothesis that there is a real difference in proportions (further discussion on this point is given in Common questions at the end of this chapter).

$$\text{SE} (p_1 - p_2) = \sqrt{\left(\frac{p_1 \times (100 - p_1)}{n_1} + \frac{p_2 \times (100 - p_2)}{n_2} \right)} \qquad (5.2)$$

Note that this is an approximate formula; the exact one would use the population proportions rather than the sample estimates.

With our appendicitis data, we have:

$$\sqrt{\left(\frac{60.8 \times 39.2}{120} + \frac{56.7 \times 43.3}{640} \right)} = 4.87$$

Thus a 95% confidence interval for the difference in percentages is:

$$4.1 - (1.96 \times 4.87) \text{ to } 4.1 + 1.96 \times 4.87$$

$$= -5.4 \text{ to } 13.6\%$$

Confidence interval for an odds ratio

The appendicitis data can be rewritten as a 2×2 table given in Table 5.1.

As discussed in Chapter 3, the odds ratio for males versus females is OR = ad/bc, which is given by $73 \times 277/363 \times 47 = 1.185$. This means that women are about 20% greater risk of being

Table 5.1 Appendicitis data.

	Cases	
	Appendicitis	**Surgical (not appendicitis)**
Females	73 (a)	363 (b)
Males	47 (c)	277 (d)
Total	120	640

an appendicitis case than men. It turns out to be easier to calculate the standard error of the $\log_e$ odds ratio. The standard error is given by:[1]

$$SE\ (\log_e OR) = \sqrt{\frac{1}{a} + \frac{1}{b} + \frac{1}{c} + \frac{1}{d}} \qquad (5.3)$$

Thus the standard error is given by:

$$\sqrt{\frac{1}{73} + \frac{1}{363} + \frac{1}{47} + \frac{1}{277}} = 0.203$$

The $\log_e$ of the odds ratio is 0.170.

Thus a 95% confidence interval for the $\log_e$ OR is given by:

$$0.170 - 1.96 \times 0.203 \text{ to } 0.170 + 1.96 \times 0.203$$

$$\text{or } -0.228 \text{ to } 0.578$$

To get a 95% confidence interval for OR, we need to take antilogs (e^x). Thus a 95% confidence interval for the odds ratio is $e^{-0.228}$ to $e^{0.578}$, which is 0.80 to 1.77. Note how this confidence interval is not symmetric about the odds ratio of 1.19, in contrast to that for a difference in proportions.

If there were no difference in the proportion of males to females for the two surgical groups, we would expect the OR to be 1. Thus if the 95% confidence interval *excludes* 1, we can say there is a significant difference between the groups. In this case, the confidence interval includes 1, in agreement with the earlier lack of significance from the statistical test.

Confidence interval for a relative risk

Consider the isoniazid trial described in Table 3.2. Using the notation of Table 3.1, the standard error of the logarithm of the relative risk is given by:[1]

$$SE\,(\log RR) = \sqrt{\frac{1}{a} - \frac{1}{a+b} + \frac{1}{c} - \frac{1}{c+d}}$$

Thus the standard error is given by:

$$SE\,(\log RR) = \sqrt{\frac{1}{21} - \frac{1}{131} + \frac{1}{11} - \frac{1}{132}} = 0.351$$

The relative risk is given by 0.52 and so the logarithm is −0.654. Thus a 95% confidence interval for the log relative risk is:

$$-0.654 - 1.96 \times 0.351 \text{ to } -0.654 + 1.96 \times 0.351$$

$$-1.42 \text{ to } 0.040$$

and so the 95% confidence interval for the relative risk is:

$$0.242 \text{ to } 1.04$$

Confidence intervals for other estimates

For any estimate, it is possible to find a confidence interval. A general method is via what is known as the *bootstrap*.[2] This method takes repeated samples, with replacement, from the original data and recalculates estimate. With a large number of samples, a range of values will be obtained, from which it will be possible to calculate where 95% (say) of them lie. In general, any worthwhile package will give a confidence interval to an estimate, and so for example *OpenEpi* gives confidence intervals for all the estimators given in Chapters 2 and 3. Different methods may give different values and one should consult the program manual for advice on which method is best under which circumstances.

Common questions

What is the difference between a reference range and a confidence interval?

There is precisely the same relationship between a reference range and a confidence interval as between the standard deviation and the standard error. The reference range refers to *individuals* and the confidence intervals to *estimates*. It is important to realize that samples are not unique. Different investigators taking samples from the same population will obtain different estimates of the population parameter, and have different 95% confidence intervals. However, we know that for 95 of every 100 investigators, the confidence interval will include the population parameter (we just don't know which ones).

If I repeated a study with the same sample size, would the new results fall in the confidence interval 95% of the time?

This is a common misperception. It ignores the fact that the new study has its own uncertainty, which needs to be included in the calculation. In fact, there is an approximately 84% chance of the new results falling within the 95% confidence interval. For further discussion, see Julious *et al.*[3]

Reading and reporting confidence intervals

- In general, confidence intervals are best restricted to the main outcome of a study, which is often a contrast (i.e. a difference) between means or percentages. There is now a great emphasis on confidence intervals in the literature, and some authors attach confidence intervals to every estimate in a paper, which is not a good idea!
- The Vancouver guidelines state "When possible, quantify findings and present them with appropriate indicators of measurement error or uncertainty (such as confidence intervals)".[4]
- To avoid confusion with negative numbers, it is best to quote a confidence interval as "a to b" rather than "a − b".

Formula appreciation

A geometric interpretation of equation (5.1) is that if SE_1 and SE_2 are sides of a triangle joined by a right angle, then SE (diff) is the length of the side of the triangle opposite the right angle. As an aside, the right angle comes about because we assume that samples 1 and 2 are *independent* (sometimes termed *orthogonal*). If they are not, for example, if some people feature in both samples 1 and 2, then formula (5.1) is no longer valid. Note that in equation (5.2), we can exchange p_1 with $1 - p_1$ and p_2 with $1 - p_2$. Thus the SE of the difference between 95% and 10% is the same as the SE for 5% and 10%, and for 95% and 90%. In formula (5.3), if *any* of a, b, c, d is small, then the SE will be large, irrespective of how big the others are.

Exercises

5.1 A count of malaria parasites in 100 fields with a 2 mm oil immersion lens gave a mean of 35 parasites per field, standard deviation 11.6 (note that, although the counts are quantitative discrete, the counts can be assumed to follow a Normal distribution because the average is large). On counting one more field, the pathologist found 52 parasites. Does this number lie outside the 95% reference range? What is the reference range?

5.2 What is the 95% confidence interval for the mean of the population from which this sample count of parasites was drawn.

5.3 In one group of 62 patients with iron deficiency anemia, the hemoglobin level was 12.2 g/dl, standard deviation 1.8 g/dl; in another group of 35 patients the hemoglobin level was 10.9 g/dl, standard deviation 2.1 g/dl. What is the difference in means and the standard error of this difference? Give an approximate 95% confidence interval for the difference.

5.4 In an obstetric hospital, 17.8% of 320 women were delivered by forceps. What is the standard error of this percentage? In another hospital in the same region, 21.2% of 185 women were delivered by forceps. What is the standard error of the difference between the percentages at this hospital and the first? What is the difference between these percentages of forceps delivery with a 95% confidence interval?

5.5 Calculate the difference in proportions (also known as the absolute risk reduction (ARR)) and a 95% confidence interval for the difference in proportions of children who died or had a shunt for the data given in Table 3.4.

5.6 For the data in Table 3.6, calculate the odds ratio for the relationship between eczema and hay fever, and find a 95% confidence interval.

References

1. Altman DG, Machin D, Bryant TN and Gardner MJ (Eds). *Statistics with Confidence*, 2nd ed. London: BMJ Publishing Group, 2000.

2. Campbell MJ. *Statistics at Square Two*. Oxford: Wiley-Blackwell, 2006.
3. Julious SA, Campbell MJ and Walters SJ. Predicting where future means will lie based on the results of the current trial. *Contemporary Clinical Trials* 2007;**28**:352–7.
4. International Committee of Medical Journal Editors. Uniform Requirements for Manuscripts Submitted to Biomedical Journals: Writing and Editing for Biomedical Publication, 2007. URL: http://www.icmje.org/

CHAPTER 6

P-values, power, type I and type II errors

We saw in Chapter 4 that the mean of a sample has a standard error, and a mean that departs by more than twice its standard error from the population mean would be expected by chance only in about 5% of samples. Likewise, the difference between the means of two samples has a standard error. We do not usually know the population mean, so we may suppose that the mean of one of our samples estimates it. The sample mean may happen to be identical with the population mean, but it more probably lies somewhere above or below the population mean, and there is a 95% chance that it is within 1.96 standard errors of it.

Null hypothesis and type I error

In comparing the mean blood pressures of the printers and the farmers, we are testing the hypothesis that the two samples came from the same population of blood pressures. The hypothesis that there is no difference between the population from which the printers' blood pressures were drawn and the population from which the farmers' blood pressures were drawn is called the *null hypothesis*.

But what do we mean by "no difference"? Chance alone will almost certainly ensure that there is some difference between the *sample* means, for they are most unlikely to be identical. Consequently, we set limits within which we shall regard the samples as not having any significant difference. If we set the limits at twice the standard error of the difference, and regard a mean outside this range as coming from another population, we shall on average be wrong about one time in 20 if the null hypothesis is in

Statistics at Square One, XIth edition. By M.J. Campbell and T.D.V. Swinscow.
Published 2009 by Blackwell Publishing, ISBN: 9781405191005.

fact true. If we do obtain a mean difference bigger than two standard errors we are faced with two choices: either an unusual event has happened or the null hypothesis is incorrect. Imagine tossing a coin 5 times and getting the same face each time. This has nearly the same probability (6.3%) as obtaining a mean difference bigger than two standard errors when the null hypothesis is true. Do we regard it as a lucky event or suspect a biased coin? If we are unwilling to believe in unlucky events, we reject the null hypothesis, which in this case is that the coin is a fair one.

To reject the null hypothesis when it is true is to make what is known as a *type I error*. The level at which a result is declared significant is known as the type I error rate, often denoted by α. We try to show that a null hypothesis is *unlikely*, not its converse (that it is likely), so a difference which is greater than the limits we have set, and which we therefore regard as "significant", makes the null hypothesis *unlikely*. However, a difference within the limits we have set, and which we therefore regard as "non-significant, does not make the hypothesis likely. To repeat an old adage, "absence of evidence is not evidence of absence".

A range of not more than two standard errors is often taken as implying "no difference" but there is nothing to stop investigators choosing a range of three standard errors (or more) if they want to reduce the chances of a type I error.

Testing for differences of two means

To find out whether the difference in blood pressure of printers and farmers could have arisen by chance, the general practitioner erects the null hypothesis that there is no significant difference between them. The question is, how many multiples of its standard error does the difference in means represent? Since the difference in means is 9.0 mmHg and its standard error is 0.805 mmHg, the answer is 9.0/0.805 = 11.2. We usually denote the ratio of an estimate to its standard error by "z", that is, $z = 11.2$. Reference to Table A (Appendix) shows that z is far beyond the figure of 3.291 standard deviations, representing a probability of 0.001 (or 1 in 1000). The probability of a difference of 11.1 standard errors or more occurring by chance is therefore exceedingly low, and correspondingly the null hypothesis that these two samples came from the same population of observations is exceedingly unlikely. The probability is known as the *P-value* and may be written $P << 0.001$.

Sometimes an investigator knows a mean from a very large number of observations and wants to compare the mean of her sample with it. We may not know the standard deviation of the large number of observations or the standard error of their mean, but this need not hinder the comparison if we can assume that the standard error of the mean of the large number of observations is near zero or at least very small in relation to the standard error of the mean of the small sample.

This is because in equation (5.1), for calculating the standard error of the difference between the two means, when n_1 is very large then SD_1^2/n_1 becomes so small as to be negligible. The formula thus reduces to

$$\sqrt{\frac{SD_2^2}{n_2}}$$

which is the same as that for standard error of the sample mean.

Consequently, we find the standard error of the mean of the sample and divide it into the difference between the means.

For example, a large number of observations have shown that the mean count of erythrocytes (measured $\times 10^{12}$ per litre) in men is 5.5. In a sample of 100 men, a mean count of 5.35 was found with standard deviation 1.1. The standard error of this mean is $SD/\sqrt{n}$, $1.1/\sqrt{100} = 0.11$. The difference between the two means is $5.5 - 5.35 = 0.15$. This difference, divided by the standard error, gives $z = 0.15/0.11 = 1.36$. This figure is well below the 5% level of 1.96 and in fact is below the 10% level of 1.645 (see Table A). We therefore conclude that the difference could have arisen by chance.

Testing for a difference in two proportions

For a significance test, we have to use a slightly different formula for the standard error of a difference in proportions to that given in the previous chapter. This one is based on the null hypothesis that both samples have a common population proportion, estimated by p.

$$SE\ (diff\ \%) = \sqrt{\left(\frac{p \times (100 - p)}{n_1} + \frac{p \times (100 - p)}{n_2}\right)}$$

From the appendicitis data referred to in Chapter 4, to obtain p we must amalgamate the two samples and calculate the percentage of women in the two combined; $100 - p$ is then the percentage of men in the two combined. The numbers in each sample are n_1 and n_2.

Number of women in the samples: $73 + 363 = 436$

Number of people in the samples: $120 + 640 = 760$

Percentage of women: $(436 \times 100)/760 = 57.4$

Percentage of men: $(324 \times 100)/760 = 42.6$

Putting these numbers in the formula, we find the standard error of the difference between the percentages is:

$$\sqrt{\left(\frac{57.4 \times 42.6}{120} + \frac{57.4 \times 42.6}{640} \right)} = 4.92$$

This is very close to the standard error estimated under the alternative hypothesis.

The difference between the percentage of women (and men) in the two samples was 4.1%. To find the probability attached to this difference, we divide it by its standard error: $z = 4.1/4.92 = 0.83$. From Table A (Appendix), we find that P is about 0.4 and so the difference between the percentages in the two samples could have been due to chance alone, as might have been expected from the confidence interval. Note that this test gives results identical to those obtained by the χ^2 test without continuity correction (described in Chapter 8).

The *P*-value

It is worth recapping this procedure, which is at the heart of statistical inference. Suppose that we have samples from two groups of subjects, and we wish to see if they could plausibly come from the same population. The first approach would be to calculate the difference between two statistics (such as the means of the two groups) and calculate the 95% confidence interval. If the two samples were from the same population, we would expect the confidence interval to include zero 95% of the time, and so if the confidence interval excludes zero we suspect that they are from a different population. The other approach is to compute the probability of getting the observed value, or *one that is more extreme*, if the null hypothesis were correct. This is the *P*-value. If this is less than

a specified level (usually 5%), then the result is declared significant and the null hypothesis is rejected. These two approaches, the
estimation and hypothesis testing approach, are complementary.
Imagine if the 95% confidence interval just captured the value
zero, what would be the P-value? A moment's thought should
convince one that it is 2.5%. This is known as a *one-sided P-value*,
because it is the probability of getting the observed result or one
bigger than it. However, the 95% confidence interval is two sided,
because it excludes not only the 2.5% above the upper limit but
also the 2.5% below the lower limit. To support the complemen-
tarity of the confidence interval approach and the null hypothesis
testing approach, most authorities double the one-sided P-value to
obtain a two-sided P-value (see below for the distinction between
one-sided and two-sided tests).

P-values, confidence intervals, and clinically important results

Simply because we have rejected a null hypothesis, this does not
mean we have found an important result. It is useful to think in
terms of a *clinically important* difference. For example, a general
practitioner might prescribe a drug which reduced blood pressure
by 10 mmHg but not one that reduced it by 1 mmHg, because the
former is clinically worthwhile. Suppose we are comparing a new
treatment with a standard and we know what a clinically important result is. Suppose we run five studies and have the results as
shown in Figure 6.1.

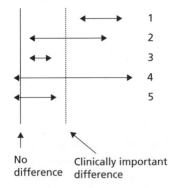

Figure 6.1 95% Confidence intervals for five studies.

In study 1, we have a statistically significant result which is also clinically important. In study 2, we have a statistically significant result, but the confidence interval suggests that it is plausible that the results are not clinically important. In study 3, the results are statistically significant but not clinically important. This could be the outcome from a very large clinical trial. In study 4, we have a result which may be clinically important, since the center of the confidence interval is bigger than the minimum clinically important difference. However it is not statistically significant. Finally, study 5 is neither statistically significant nor clinically important. This may be a useful result if one was interested in proving two treatments were equivalent.

Alternative hypothesis and type II error

It is important to realize that when we are comparing two groups, a non-significant result does not mean that we have proved the two samples come from the same population—it simply means that we have failed to prove that they do *not* come from the same population. When planning studies, it is useful to think of what differences are likely to arise between the two groups, or what would be clinically worthwhile; for example, what do we expect to be the improved benefit from a new treatment in a clinical trial? This leads to a *study hypothesis*, which is a difference we would like to demonstrate. To contrast the study hypothesis with the null hypothesis, it is often called the *alternative hypothesis*. If we do not reject the null hypothesis when in fact there is a difference between the groups, we make what is known as a *type II error*. The type II error rate is often denoted as β. The *power* of a study is defined as $1 - \beta$ and is the probability of rejecting the null hypothesis when it is false. The most common reason for type II errors is that the study is too small.

The relationship between type I and type II errors is shown in Table 6.1. One has to imagine a series of cases, in some of which the null hypothesis is true and in some of which it is false. In either situation we carry out a significance test, which sometimes is significant and sometimes not.

The concept of power is *only* relevant when a study is being planned (see Chapter 13 for sample size calculations). After a study has been completed, we wish to make statements not about hypothetical alternative hypotheses but about the data, and the way to do this is with estimates and confidence intervals.

Table 6.1 Relationship between type I and type II errors.

		Null hypothesis	
		False	True
Test result	Significant	Power	Type I error
	Not significant	Type II error	

Common questions

Why is the standard error used for calculating a confidence interval for the difference in two proportions different from the standard error used for calculating the significance?

For nominal variables, the standard deviation is not independent of the mean. If we suppose that a nominal variable simply takes the value 0 or 1, then the mean is simply the proportion of 1's and the standard deviation is directly dependent on the mean, being largest when the mean is 0.5. The null and alternative hypotheses are hypotheses about means, either that they are the same (null) or different (alternative). Thus for nominal variables, the standard deviations (and thus the standard errors) will also be different for the null and alternative hypotheses. For a confidence interval, the alternative hypothesis is assumed to be true, whereas for a significance test the null hypothesis is assumed to be true. In general, the difference in the values of the two methods of calculating the standard errors is likely to be small, and use of either would lead to the same inferences. The reason this is mentioned here is that there is a close connection between the test of significance described in this chapter and the χ^2 test described in Chapter 8. The difference in the arithmetic for the significance test, and that for calculating the confidence interval, could lead some readers to believe that they are unrelated, whereas in fact they are complementary. The problem does not arise with continuous variables, where the standard deviation is usually assumed independent of the mean, and is also assumed to be the same value under both the null and alternative hypotheses.

It is worth pointing out that the formula for calculating the standard error of an estimate is not necessarily unique; it depends on underlying assumptions, and so different assumptions or study designs will lead to different estimates for standard errors for data sets that might be numerically identical.

Why is the *P*-value not the probability that the null hypothesis is true?

A moment's reflection should convince you that the *P*-value could not be the probability that the null hypothesis is true. Suppose we got exactly the same value for the mean in two samples (if the samples were small and the observations coarsely rounded this would not be uncommon; the difference between the means is zero). The probability of getting the observed result (zero) or a result more extreme (a result that is either positive or negative) is unity—that is, we can be certain that we must obtain a result which is positive, negative, or zero. However, we can never be certain that the null hypothesis is true, especially with small samples, so clearly the statement that the *P*-value is the probability that the null hypothesis is true is in error. We can think of it as a measure of the strength of evidence against the null hypothesis, but since it is critically dependent on the sample size we should not compare *P*-values to argue that a difference found in one group is more "significant" than a difference found in another.

Why is 5% usually used as the level by which results are deemed "significant"

There are a number of different suggestions as to why 5% has achieved such iconic status. The most prosaic is that it nearly corresponds to a difference of two standard errors. Another derives from the way the great statistician RA Fisher tabulated *P*-values. However, a simple class experiment is to toss a coin repeatedly and tell the class that the outcome is a "head" irrespective of the true outcome. They usually start to disbelieve you after 4 or 5 heads. Since the probability of 4 heads is 1/16 and 5 is 1/32, the "person in the street" generally starts to disbelieve results which have a probability in this range. However, there are reasons to suggest that a smaller threshold may be appropriate (see below).

What is the difference between a one-sided and a two-sided test?

Consider a test to compare the population means of two groups A and B. A one-sided test considers as an alternative hypothesis that mean A is greater than mean B. A two-sided test considers as an alternative that mean A is either greater *or* less than B. Since the one-sided test requires a stronger assumption, it is more powerful. However, it leaves one in a dilemma if the *observed* mean of A is much less than the observed mean of B. In theory, one cannot abandon the one-sided alternative hypothesis and choose a two-sided one instead. Since, in most cases, we are genuinely uncertain as to which direction to choose, two-sided tests are almost universal. The main exception may be when one is trying to show two treatments are *equivalent*, for example, lumpectomy compared with radical mastectomy for breast cancer. Then the question is whether lumpectomy is *worse* for survival, and we are not worried if it might be better. Note that at the beginning of this chapter, we referred to the probability of the same side of a coin turning up after five tosses as 6.3%, whereas just earlier we gave the probability of 5 heads as $1/32 = 3.1\%$. In the former case, we were not concerned whether we saw a head or a tail and so used a two-tailed test, whereas in the latter case we specified a head and so used a one-tailed test.

Are there other methods of statistical inference?

We reiterate the definition of a *P*-value: the probability of getting an observed result, or one more extreme, if the null hypothesis were true. As stated above, it is not the probability of the null hypothesis being true; the null hypothesis is assumed true in this case. If *D* represents data and *H* the null hypothesis, the *P*-value is $P(D|H)$ (probability of the data *given* the hypothesis) and not $P(H|D)$ (probability of the hypothesis *given* the data). To get from one to the other we need Bayes' theorem. This states that $P(H|D)$ is proportional to $P(D|H) \times P(H)$. The term $P(H)$ is termed the *prior distribution* and measures our prior beliefs about the distribution of the treatment response (there are difficulties about specifying this but the distribution can be based on earlier studies and clinical judgement). The *posterior* distribution is the measure of our beliefs about the distribution of the treatment response after we have collected the data. This combines both our prior beliefs and the observed data from the current trial. We can then use the posterior distribution to give an estimate of the likely treatment response with a *credibility interval* to give a range of plausible values. A Bayesian credibility interval is analogous to a frequentist confidence interval. Provided one has a sufficient quantity of data, one would like the data to inform our beliefs after the study, and the prior distribution to have little effect. We can also set what is known as a "vague" or non-informative prior distribution. There may be difficulties formulating these, but essentially they are such that we will only rely on the observed data for inference. In this case, the *one-sided P*-value *can* be interpreted as a probability about the null hypothesis (Burton *et al.*[1]). If by chance two means are found to be identical, then the one-sided *P*-value is 0.5. A vague prior distribution would chosen so that initially we have no prejudice about where the difference in means is to be. With $P = 0.5$, we say that the most likely hypothesis is the null one. However, there is a fifty-fifty chance that any other hypothesis could be true.

However, suppose one had results from two clinical trials. One was a test of aspirin versus placebo for the treatment of headache, and we found $P = 0.04$. The other was a test of a homeopathic remedy versus control for ill health, and out of several outcomes, headache also had a *P*-value of 0.04. Does one give equal weight to these two *P*-values? In general the answer would be no; one has a stronger prior belief about the efficacy of aspirin. Goodman suggested using what are known as Bayes factors in these cases.[2] He argues that what is needed is an inferential index that doesn't simply accept or reject a hypothesis, but tells us how far we have come when we have collected data. We can use Bayes factors to convert prior *odds of* competing hypotheses to posterior odds. Assuming a Normal outcome the strongest Bayes factor is given by $\exp(-z^2/2)$. Thus from Table A (Appendix), if $P = 0.05$, $z = 1.96$, then the Bayes factor is 0.15. Similarly the Bayes factor corresponding to $P = 0.01$ is 0.04. Suppose we thought there was a fifty-fifty chance of the null hypothesis being true. This is an odds of 1 and so if $P = 0.05$ the smallest posterior odds are 0.15, or a probability of $0.15/(1 + 0.15) = 0.13$. If $P = 0.01$ then the posterior probability becomes 0.035. These results are quite surprising. A 50% chance of the null hypothesis being true is not high, and yet with $P = 0.05$ there is still at least a 13% chance of the null hypothesis being true. It is only when $P = 0.01$ does the posterior probability drop below 1 in 20. This led Sterne and Smith[3] to suggest that $P = 0.05$ is only moderate evidence against the null hypothesis; $P = 0.01$ is moderate to strong and $P = 0.001$ is strong to very strong.

Reading and reporting *P*-values

- If possible present a precise *P*-value (e.g. $P = 0.031$) rather than a range such as $0.02 < P < 0.05$.

- Do NOT report values of $P > 0.05$ as "n.s.". Instead give the exact P-value.
- It is unnecessary to go beyond two significant figures for P-values, and for small values $P < 0.001$ will usually suffice.
- Some computer programs give small values as $P = 0.000$. Report $P < 0.001$ instead.
- Do not use phrases such as "tending toward significance" for P-values just over 0.05. Quote the actual P-value and perhaps use other corroborating details (biological plausibility, direction of the result, other people's results) to decide whether or not to reject the null hypothesis. Remember that the 0.05 level is not an absolute barrier to deciding to reject or not. However, also remember that other people may have differing beliefs and so not accept your decision.
- Beware P-values from exploratory studies (Chapter 13) which do not have a limited number of prior null hypotheses. They may be the result of 'data-dredging' which involves testing a large number of hypotheses to find the most 'significant' result.

Exercises

6.1 A clinical trial to compare a mouthwash against a control found a difference in plaque score after 1 year of 1.1 units, $P = 0.006$ (two sided). The following are true or false.
   (a) The probability that the null hypothesis is true is 0.006.
   (b) If the null hypothesis were true, the probability of getting an observed result of 1.1 or greater is 0.003.
   (c) The alternative hypothesis is a mean difference of 1.1.
   (d) The probability of the alternative hypothesis being true is 0.994.
   (e) The probability that the true mean is 1.1 units is 95%.

6.2 The 95% confidence interval for the mean difference in scores was found to be (0.3 to 1.9 units). The following are true or false.
   (a) We are 95% sure that the true mean lies between 0.3 and 1.9 units.
   (b) If the study were repeated many times, the 95% confidence interval would include the true mean 95% of the time.
   (c) If we repeated the study with the same sample size, we would expect the mean difference to be within 0.3 to 1.9 units 95% of the time.

(d) The study is clinically important.

(e) The power of the study is greater than 80%.

6.3 What is the *P*-value associated with the results given in exercise 5.3?

References

1. Burton PR, Gurrin LC and Campbell MJ. Clinical significance not statistical significance: a simple Bayesian alternative to *p*-values. *J Epidemiol Community Health* 1998;**52**:318–23.
2. Goodman SN. Of *P*-values and Bayes: a modest proposal. *Epidemiology* 2001;**12**:295–7.
3. Sterne JAC and Smith GD. Sifting the evidence—what's wrong with significance tests? *BMJ* 2001;**322**:226–31.

CHAPTER 7
The *t* tests

Previously we have considered how to test the null hypothesis that there is no difference between the mean of a sample and the population mean, and no difference between the means of two samples. We obtained the difference between the means by subtraction, and then divided this difference by the standard error of the difference. If the difference is 1.96 times its standard error, or more, it is likely to occur by chance with a frequency of only 1 in 20, or less.

With small samples, where more chance variation must be allowed for, these ratios are not entirely accurate because the uncertainty in estimating the standard error has been ignored. Some modification of the procedure of dividing the difference by its standard error is needed, and the technique to use is the *t* test. Its foundations were laid by WS Gosset, writing under the pseudonym "Student" so that it is sometimes known as Student's *t* test. The procedure does not differ greatly from the one used for large samples, but is preferable when the number of observations is less than 60, and certainly when they amount to 30 or less.

The application of the *t* distribution to the following four types of problem will now be considered:

1 The calculation of a confidence interval for a sample mean.
2 The mean and standard deviation of a sample are calculated and a value is postulated for the mean of the population. How significantly does the sample mean differ from the postulated population mean?
3 The means and standard deviations of two samples are calculated. Could both samples have been taken from the same population?

Statistics at Square One, XIth edition. By M.J. Campbell and T.D.V. Swinscow.
Published 2009 by Blackwell Publishing, ISBN: 9781405191005.

4 Paired observations are made on two samples (or in succession on one sample). What is the significance of the difference between the means of the two sets of observations?

In each case the problem is essentially the same—namely, to establish multiples of standard errors to which probabilities can be attached. These multiples are the number of times a difference can be divided by its standard error. We have seen that with large samples 1.96 times the standard error has a probability of 5% or less, and 2.576 times the standard error a probability of 1% or less (Table A in the Appendix). With small samples, these multiples are larger, and the smaller the sample the larger they become.

Confidence interval for the mean from a small sample

A rare congenital disease, Everley's syndrome, generally causes a reduction in concentration of blood sodium. This is thought to provide a useful diagnostic sign as well as a clue to the efficacy of treatment. Little is known about the subject, but the director of a dermatological department in a London teaching hospital is known to be interested in the disease and has seen more cases than anyone else. Even so, he has seen only 18. The patients were all aged between 20 and 44.

The mean blood sodium concentration of these 18 cases was 115 mmol/l, with standard deviation of 12 mmol/l. Assuming that blood sodium concentration is Normally distributed, what is the 95% confidence interval within which the mean of the total population of such cases may be expected to lie?

The data are set out as follows:

Number of observations	18
Mean blood sodium concentration	115 mmol/l
Standard deviation	12 mmo1/l
Standard error of mean	$SD/\sqrt{n} = 12/\sqrt{18} = 2.83$ mmol/l

To find the 95% confidence interval above and below the mean, we now have to find a multiple of the standard error. In large samples we have seen that the multiple is 1.96 (Chapter 5). The difficulty is that in theory the standard deviation should be already known. When the standard deviation is estimated from the data, the Normal distribution is only an approximation, even when the original data are Normally distributed. The approximation becomes poorer for small samples and the correct distribution is known as the t distribution. To find the t-value associated with say, a probability of 0.05, we use the TINV function in OpenOffice Calc. As the sample becomes smaller, t becomes larger for any particular level of probability. Conversely, as the sample becomes larger, t becomes smaller and approaches the Normal values given in Table A (Appendix), reaching them for infinitely large samples.

Since the size of the sample influences the value of t, the size of the sample is taken into account in relating the value of t to a probability. Rather than the sample size we enter the "degrees of freedom". The use of these was noted in the calculation of the standard deviation (Chapter 2). In practice, the degrees of freedom for a single mean amount to one less than the number of observations in the sample. With these data we have $18 - 1 = 17$ d.f. This is because only 17 observations plus the total number of observations are needed to specify the sample, the 18th being determined by subtraction.

To find the number by which we must multiply the standard error to give the 95% confidence interval, we find the 5% point of t with 17 d.f. from OpenOffice Calc to discover the number 2.110. The 95% confidence intervals of the mean are now set as follows:

$$\text{Mean} - 2.110\ \text{SE to Mean} + 2.110\ \text{SE}$$

which gives us:

$$115 - (2.110 \times 2.83) \text{ to } 115 + 2.110 \times 2.83$$

$$\text{or } 109.03 \text{ to } 120.97\,\text{mmol/l}$$

We may then say, with a 95% chance of being correct, that the range 109.03 to 120.97 mmol/l includes the population mean. Likewise for a 99% confidence interval the t-value is 2.898: which gives a 99% confidence interval of:

$$115 - (2.898 \times 2.83) \text{ to } 115 + (2.898 \times 2.83)$$

$$\text{or } 106.80 \text{ to } 123.20\,\text{mmol/l}$$

Difference of sample mean from population mean (one sample *t* test)

Estimations of plasma calcium concentration in the 18 patients with Everley's syndrome gave a mean of 3.2 mmol/l, with standard deviation 1.1. Previous experience from a number of investigations and published reports had shown that the mean was commonly close to 2.5 mmol/l in healthy people aged 20–44, the age range of the patients. Is the mean in these patients abnormally high?

The assumptions are:

- Data are representative of people with Everley's syndrome (in this case we have a *convenience* sample).
- Data are quantitative and plausibly Normally distributed.
- Data are independent of each other. This assumption is most important. In general, repeated measurements on the same individual are not independent. If we had 18 measures of plasma calcium on 15 patients, then we have only 15 independent observations.

We set the figures out as follows:

Mean of general population, μ	2.5 mmol/l
Mean of sample, $\bar{x}$	3.2 mmol/l
Standard deviation of sample, SD	1.1 mmol/l
Standard error of sample mean, SD/$\sqrt{n}$ = 1.1/$\sqrt{18}$	0.26 mmo1/l
Difference between means $\mu - \bar{x}$ = 2.5 − 3.2	−0.7 mmol/l

t = difference between means divided by standard error of sample mean

$$t = \frac{\mu - \bar{x}}{\text{SD}/\sqrt{n}} = \frac{-0.7}{0.26} = -2.69$$

Degrees of freedom, $n - 1 = 18 - 1 = 17$.

Using OpenOffice Calc TDIST, we find $P = 0.015$ (two sided). It is therefore unlikely that the sample with mean 3.2 came from the population with mean 2.5, and we may conclude that the sample mean is, at least statistically, unusually high. Whether it should be regarded clinically as abnormally high is something that needs to be considered separately by the physician in charge of that case.

Difference between means of two samples

Here we apply a modified procedure for finding the standard error of the difference between two means and testing the size of the difference by this standard error (see Chapter 5 for large samples). For large samples we used the standard deviation of each sample, computed separately, to calculate the standard error of the difference between the means. For small samples we calculate a combined standard deviation for the two samples. The following example illustrates the procedure.

The addition of bran to the diet has been reported to benefit patients with diverticulosis. Several different bran preparations are available, and a clinician wants to test the efficacy of two of them on patients, since favorable claims have been made for each. Among the consequences of administering bran that requires testing is the transit time through the alimentary canal. Does it differ in the two groups of patients taking these two preparations?

The null hypothesis is that the two groups come from the same population. By random allocation the clinician selects two groups of patients aged 40–64 with diverticulosis of comparable severity. Sample 1 contains 15 patients who are given treatment A, and sample 2 contains 12 patients who are given treatment B. The transit times of food through the gut are measured by a standard technique with marked pellets and the results are recorded, in order of increasing time, in Table 7.1.

Table 7.1 Transit times of marker pellets through the alimentary canal of patients with diverticulosis on two types of treatment: unpaired comparison.

	Transit times (h)	
	Sample 1 (treatment A)	Sample 2 (treatment B)
	44	52
	51	64
	52	68
	55	74
	60	79
	62	83
	66	84
	68	88
	69	95
	71	97
	71	101
	76	116
	82	
	91	
	108	
Total	1026	1001
Mean	68.40	83.42

The assumptions are:
- The two samples come from distributions that may differ in their mean value, but not in the standard deviation.
- The observations are independent of each other.
- The data are quantitative and plausibly Normally distributed. (Note in the case of a randomized trial, this last assumption is less critical, see Common questions.)

These data are shown in Figure 7.1. The assumptions of approximate Normality and equality of variance are satisfied. The design suggests that the observations are indeed independent. Since it is possible for the difference in mean transit times for A − B to be positive or negative, we will employ a two-sided test.

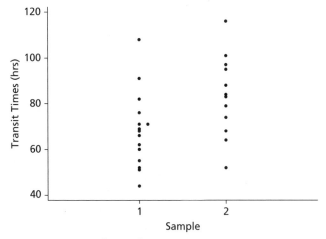

Figure 7.1 Transit times for two bran preparations

With treatment A, the mean transit time was 68.40 h and with treatment B 83.42 h. What is the significance of the difference, 15.02 h?

Find the pooled variance:

$$s_p^2 = \frac{(n_1 - 1)s_1^2 + (n_2 - 1)s_2^2}{n_1 + n_2 - 2}$$

The standard error of the difference between the means is:

$$\mathrm{SE}(\bar{x}_1 - \bar{x}_2) = s_p \sqrt{\left(\frac{1}{n_1} + \frac{1}{n_2} \right)}$$

When the difference between the means is divided by this standard error, the result is t. Thus,

$$t = \frac{(\bar{x}_1 - \bar{x}_2)}{\sqrt{\left(\dfrac{s_p^2}{n_1} + \dfrac{s_p^2}{n_2}\right)}}$$

The test has $(n_1 - 1) + (n_2 - 1)$ degrees of freedom.

For the transit times of Table 7.1,

Treatment A $n_1 = 15,$ $\bar{x}_1 = 68.40,$ $s_1 = 16.474$

Treatment B $n_2 = 12,$ $\bar{x}_2 = 83.42,$ $s_2 = 17.635$

$$s_p^2 = \frac{14 \times 271.3927 + 11 \times 310.9932}{(15-1) + (12-1)} = 288.82$$

$$SE(\bar{x}_1 - \bar{x}_2) = \sqrt{(288.82/15 + 288.82/12)} = 6.582$$

$$t = \frac{83.42 - 68.40}{6.582} = 2.282$$

OpenOffice Calc TDIST (two sided) shows that with 25 degrees of freedom (i.e. $(15 - 1) + (12 - 1)$), $P = 0.02$.

This degree of probability is smaller than the conventional level of 5%. The null hypothesis that there is no difference between the means is therefore somewhat unlikely.

A 95% confidence interval is given by:

$$\bar{x}_1 - \bar{x}_2 \pm t(n_1 + n_2 - 2) \times SE$$

OpenOffice Calc TINV(0.05;25) = 2.06

The 95% confidence interval becomes:

$$83.42 - 68.40 \pm 2.06 \times 6.582$$

$$15.02 - 13.56 \text{ to } 15.02 + 13.56$$

$$\text{or } 1.46 \text{ to } 28.58\,\text{h.}$$

These results are also given using OpenStat in Chapter 14.

Unequal standard deviations

If the standard deviations in the two groups are markedly different, for example if the ratio of the larger to the smaller is greater
than two, then one of the assumptions of the *t* test (that the two
samples come from populations with the same standard deviation) is unlikely to hold. An approximate test, due to Sattherwaite
and described by Armitage *et al.*,[1] which allows for unequal standard deviations, is described below. Another version of this test is
known as Welch test.

Rather than use the pooled estimate of variance, compute:

$$SE(\bar{x}_1 - \bar{x}_2) = \sqrt{\left(\frac{s_1^2}{n_1} + \frac{s_2^2}{n_2}\right)}$$

This is the large sample estimate given in equation (5.1), and is anal-
ogous to calculating the standard error of the difference in two proportions under the alternative hypothesis as described in Chapter 6.

We now compute

$$d = \frac{(\bar{x}_1 - \bar{x}_2)}{SE\ (\bar{x}_1 - \bar{x}_2)}$$

We then test this using a *t* statistic, in which the degrees of freedom are:

$$d.f. = \frac{(s_1^2/n_1 + s_2^2/n_2)^2}{[(s_1^2/n_1)^2/(n_1 - 1)] + [(s_2^2/n_2)^2/(n_2 - 1)]} \tag{7.1}$$

This is a complicated formula but luckily is implemented in
OpenStat where the results are shown in Chapter 14. The unequal
variance *t* test tends to be less powerful (i.e. slightly less likely to
give a significant result) than the usual *t* test if the variances are
in fact the same, since it uses fewer assumptions. It should not
be used indiscriminately because, if the standard deviations are
different, how can we interpret a non-significant difference in
means, for example? Often a better strategy is to try a data transformation, such as taking logarithms as described in Chapter 2.
Transformations that render distributions closer to Normality often
also make the standard deviations similar. If a log transformation is
successful, use the usual *t* test on the logged data.

We find in this case that SE = 6.632, d = 2.26, and d.f. = 22.9, or approximately 23. OpenOffice Calc gives P = 0.034, very close to that given by the equal variance test. This might be expected, because the standard deviations in the original data set are very similar, and so using the unequal variances t test gives very similar results to the t test which assumes equal variances. It can also be shown that if the numbers of observations in each group are similar, the usual t test is quite robust.

Difference between means of paired samples (paired t test)

When the effects of two alternative treatments or experiments are compared, for example in crossover trials, randomized trials in which randomization is between matched pairs, or matched case–control studies (see Chapter 13), it is sometimes possible to make comparisons in pairs. Matching controls for the matched variables can lead to a more powerful study.

The test is derived from the single sample t test, using the following assumptions.

1 The data are quantitative.
2 The distribution of the *differences* (not the original data) is plausibly Normal.
3 The differences are independent of each other.

The first case to consider is when each member of the sample acts as his own control. Whether treatment A or treatment B is given first or second to each member of the sample should be determined by the use of the table of random numbers (Appendix, Table B). In this way any effect of one treatment on the other, even indirectly through the patient's attitude to treatment, for instance, can be minimized. Occasionally it is possible to give both treatments simultaneously, as in the treatment of a skin disease by applying a remedy to the skin on opposite sides of the body.

Let us use as an example the studies of bran in the treatment of diverticulosis discussed earlier. The clinician wonders whether transit time would be shorter if bran is given in the same dosage in three meals during the day (treatment A) or in one meal (treatment B). A random sample of patients with disease of comparable severity and aged 20–44 is chosen and the two treatments administered on two successive occasions, the order of the treatments also being determined from the table of random numbers. The alimentary transit

Table 7.2 Transit times of marker pellets through the alimentary canal of 12 patients with diverticulosis on two types of treatment.

Patient	Transit times (h)		Difference A − B
	Treatment A	Treatment B	
1	63	55	8
2	54	62	−8
3	79	108	−29
4	68	77	−9
5	87	83	4
6	84	78	6
7	92	79	13
8	57	94	−37
9	66	69	−3
10	53	66	−13
11	76	72	4
12	63	77	−14
Total	842	920	−78
Mean	70.17	76.67	−6.5

times and the differences for each pair of treatments are set out in Table 7.2.

In calculating t on the paired observations, we work with the difference, d, between the members of each pair. Our first task is to find the mean of the differences between the observations and then the standard error of the mean, proceeding as follows:

Find the mean of the differences, $\bar{d}$.

Find the standard deviation of the differences, SD.

Calculate the standard error of the mean $\mathrm{SE}(\bar{d}) = \mathrm{SD}/\sqrt{n}$.

To calculate t, divide the mean of the differences by the standard error of the mean

$$t = \frac{\bar{d}}{\mathrm{SE}(\bar{d})}$$

For the data from Table 7.2, we have $\bar{d} = -6.5$, SD = 15.1, and $\mathrm{SE}(\bar{d}) = 4.37$. Thus,

$$t = -6.5/4.37 = -1.487$$

Using OpenOffice Calc TDIST with 11 degrees of freedom $(n - 1)$ and ignoring the minus sign, we find $P = 0.165$. The null hypothesis is that there is no difference between the mean transit times on these two forms of treatment. From our calculations, it is *not* disproved. However, this does not mean that the two treatments are equivalent. To help us decide this we calculate the confidence interval.

A 95% confidence interval for the mean difference is given by:

$$\bar{d} \pm t_{n-1}\text{SE}(\bar{d})$$

In this case at $P = 0.05$ with 11 d.f. $t = 2.201$ (from OpenOffice Calc TINV) and so the 95% confidence interval is:

$$-6.5 - 2.201 \times 4.37 \text{ to } -6.5 + 2.201 \times 4.37\,\text{h}$$

$$\text{or } -16.1 \text{ to } 3.1\,\text{h}$$

This interval is quite wide, so that, even though it contains zero, we cannot really conclude that the two preparations are equivalent, and should look to a larger study.

The second case of a paired comparison to consider is when two samples are chosen and each member of sample 1 is paired with one member of sample 2, as in a matched case–control study. As the aim is to test the difference, if any, between two types of treatment, the choice of members for each pair is designed to make them as alike as possible. The more alike they are, the more apparent will be any differences due to treatment, because they will not be confused with differences in the results caused by disparities between members of the pair. The likeness within the pairs applies to attributes relating to the study in question. For instance, in a test for a drug reducing blood pressure, the color of the patients' eyes would probably be irrelevant, but their resting diastolic blood pressure could well provide a basis for selecting the pairs. Another (perhaps related) basis is the prognosis for the disease in patients: in general, patients with a similar prognosis are best paired. Whatever criteria are chosen, it is essential that the pairs are constructed before the treatment is given, for the pairing must be uninfluenced by knowledge of the effects of treatment.

Further methods

Suppose we had a parallel clinical trial with more than two treatment arms. It is not valid to compare each treatment with each other treatment using *t* tests because the overall type I error rate *a* will be bigger than the conventional level set for each individual test. A method of controlling for this is to use a *one way analysis of variance* and is discussed in *Statistics at Square Two*.

Common questions

Should I test my data for Normality before using the *t* test?

It would seem logical that, because the *t* test assumes Normality, one should test for Normality first. The problem is that the test for Normality is dependent on the sample size. With a small sample a non-significant result does not mean that the data come from a Normal distribution. On the other hand, with a large sample, a significant result does not mean that we could not use the *t* test, because the *t* test is *robust* to moderate departures from Normality— that is, the *P*-value obtained can be validly interpreted. There is something illogical about using one significance test conditional on the results of another significance test. In general it is a matter of knowing and looking at the data. One can "eyeball" the data and if the distributions are not extremely skewed, and particularly if (for the two sample *t* test) the numbers of observations are similar in the two groups, then the *t* test will be valid. The main problem is often that outliers will inflate the standard deviations and render the test less sensitive. Also, it is not generally appreciated that if the data originate from a randomized controlled trial, then the process of randomization will ensure the validity of the *t* test, irrespective of the original distribution of the data. This is because the *P*-values from what is known as the randomization test, which is a non-parametric test (see Chapter 10) and does not require the assumption of Normality, can be shown to be close to those of the *t* test.[2] (RA Fisher[3] wrote " ...the physical act of randomization...affords the means in respect of any particular body of data, of examining the wider hypothesis in which no normality of distribution is implied".)

Should I test for equality of the standard deviations before using the usual *t* test?

The same argument prevails here as for the previous question about Normality. The test for equality of variances is dependent on the sample size. A rule of thumb is that if the ratio of the larger to smaller standard deviation is greater than two, then the unequal variance test should be used. In view of the fact that when the variances are similar, the equal variance and unequal variance *t* test tend to agree, there is a good argument for always doing the unequal variance test. With a computer one can easily do both the equal and unequal variance *t* test and see if the answers differ.

Why should I use a paired test if my data are paired? What happens if I don't?

Pairing provides information about an experiment, and the more information that can be provided in the analysis the more sensitive the test. One of the major sources of variability is between subjects variability. By repeating measures within subjects, each subject acts as their own control, and the between subjects variability is removed. In general this means that if there is a true difference between the pairs, the paired test is more likely to pick it up: it is more powerful. When the pairs are generated by matching the matching criteria may not be important. In this case, the paired and unpaired tests should give similar results.

Formula appreciation

In formula (7.1), the only real effect occurs when there are unequal sample sizes in the two groups as well as unequal variances. If the sample sizes are approximately similar then again the *t* test is quite robust.

Reading and reporting *t* tests

- Lack of Normality is not too much of a worry because, as stated earlier, the *t* test is remarkably robust to lack of Normality, particularly if the numbers of data points are similar in the two groups. However, one should check that the data are independent, and that the variances are similar in the two groups.
- Always report the *t* statistic, its degrees of freedom, and *P*-value. Also give the estimate and confidence interval. Thus, the transit time study for a two sample *t* test would be reported as $t = 2.28$, d.f. $= 25$, $P = 0.031$, difference in means 15.02 h, 95% CI 1.46 to 28.58 h.

Exercises

7.1 In 22 patients with an unusual liver disease, the plasma alkaline phosphatase was found by a certain laboratory to have a mean value of 39 King–Armstrong units, standard deviation 3.4 units. What is the 95% confidence interval within which the mean of the population of such cases whose specimens come to the same laboratory may be expected to lie?

7.2 In the 18 patients with Everley's syndrome, the mean level of plasma phosphate was 1.7 mmol/l, standard deviation 0.8. If the mean level in the general population is taken as 1.2 mmol/l, what is the significance of the difference between that mean and the mean of these 18 patients?

7.3 In two wards for elderly women in a geriatric hospital, the following levels of hemoglobin (g/dl) were found:

Ward A: 12.2, 11.1, 14.0, 11.3, 10.8, 12.5, 12.2, 11.9, 13.6, 12.7, 13.4, 13.7;

Ward B: 11.9, 10.7, 12.3, 13.9, 11.1, 11.2, 13.3, 11.4, 12.0, 11.1.

What is the difference between the mean levels in the two wards, and what is its significance? What is the 95% confidence interval for the difference in treatments?

7.4 A new treatment for varicose ulcer is compared with a standard treatment on 10 matched pairs of patients, where treatment between pairs is decided using random numbers. The outcome is the number of days from start of treatment to healing of ulcer. One doctor is responsible for treatment and a second doctor assesses healing without knowing which treatment each patient had. The following treatment times were recorded:

Standard treatment: 35, 104, 27, 53, 72, 64, 97, 121, 86, 41 days;

New treatment: 27, 52, 46, 33, 37, 82, 51, 92, 68, 62 days.

What are the mean difference in the healing time, the value of *t*, the number of degrees of freedom, and the probability? What is the 95% confidence interval for the difference?

References

1. Armitage P, Berry G and Matthews JNS. *Statistical Methods in Medical Research*, 4th ed. Oxford: Wiley-Blackwell, 2002:112–3.

2. David HA. The beginnings of randomization tests. *Am Stat* 2008;**62**:70–2.

3. Fisher RA. *The Design of Experiments*. Edinburgh: Oliver and Boyd, 1935.

CHAPTER 8

The χ^2 tests

The distribution of a categorical variable in a sample often needs to be compared with the distribution of a categorical variable in another sample. For example, over a period of 2 years, a psychiatrist has classified by socioeconomic class the women aged 20–64 admitted to her unit suffering from self-poisoning—sample A. At the same time she has likewise classified the women of similar age admitted to a gastroenterological unit in the same hospital—sample B. She has employed the Registrar General's five socioeconomic classes, and generally classified the women by reference to their father's or husband's occupation. The results are set out in Table 8.1.

Table 8.1 Distribution by socioeconomic class of patients admitted to self-poisoning (sample A) and gastroenterological (sample B) units.

Socioeconomic class	Samples			Proportion in Group A
	A	B	Total	
	a	b	$n = a + b$	$p = a/n$
I	17	5	22	0.77
II	25	21	46	0.54
III	39	34	73	0.53
IV	42	49	91	0.46
V	32	25	57	0.56
Total	155	134	289	

Statistics at Square One, XIth edition. By M.J. Campbell and T.D.V. Swinscow.
Published 2009 by Blackwell Publishing, ISBN: 9781405191005.

The psychiatrist wants to investigate whether the distribution of the patients by social class differed in these two units. She therefore erects the null hypothesis that there is no difference between the two distributions. This is what is tested by the chi-squared (χ^2) test (pronounced with a hard ch as in "sky"). By default, all (χ^2) tests are two sided.

It is important to emphasize here that χ^2 tests may be carried out for this purpose only on the *actual numbers* of occurrences, *not* on percentages, proportions, means of observations, or other derived statistics. Note, we distinguish here the Greek (χ^2) for the test and the distribution and the Roman (X^2) for the calculated statistic, which is what is obtained from the test.

The χ^2 test is carried out in the following steps:

For each observed number (O) in the table find an "expected" number (E); this procedure is discussed below.

Subtract each expected number from each observed number	$O - E$
Square the difference	$(O - E)^2$
Divide the squares so obtained for each cell of the table by the expected number for that cell	$(O - E)^2/E$

X^2 is the sum of $(O - E)^2/E$.

To calculate the expected number for each cell of the table, consider the null hypothesis, which in this case is that the numbers in each cell are proportionately the same in sample A as they are in sample B. We therefore construct a parallel table in which the proportions are exactly the same for both samples. This has been done in columns (2) and (3) of Table 8.2.

Table 8.2 Calculation of the χ^2 test on figures in Table 8.1.

Class (I)	Expected numbers		$O - E$		$(O - E)^2/E$	
	A (2)	B (3)	A (4)	B (5)	A (6)	B (7)
I	11.80	10.20	5.20	−5.20	2.292	2.651
II	24.67	21.33	0.33	−0.33	0.004	0.005
III	39.15	33.85	−0.15	0.15	0.001	0.001
IV	48.81	42.19	−6.81	6.81	0.950	1.099
V	30.57	26.43	1.43	−1.43	0.067	0.077
Total	155.00	134.00	0	0	3.314	3.833

$X^2 = 3.314 + 3.833 = 7.147$, d.f. = $P = 0.13$.

The proportions are obtained from the totals column in Table 8.1 and are applied to the totals row. For instance, in Table 8.2, column (2), 11.80 = (22/289) × 155; 24.67 = (46/289) × 155; in column (3), 10.20 = (22/289) × 134; 21.33 = (46/289) × 134, and so on.

Thus by simple proportions from the totals, we find an expected number to match each observed number. The sum of the expected numbers for each sample must equal the sum of the observed numbers for each sample, which is a useful check. We now subtract each expected number from its corresponding observed number.

The results are given in columns (4) and (5) of Table 8.2. Here two points may be noted.

1 The sum of these differences always equals zero in each column.
2 Each difference for sample A is matched by the same figure, but with opposite sign, for sample B.

Again these are useful checks.

The figures in columns (4) and (5) are then each squared and divided by the corresponding expected numbers in columns (2) and (3). The results are given in columns (6) and (7). Finally these results, $(O - E)^2/E$, are added. The sum of them is X^2.

Having obtained a value for $X^2 = \Sigma[(O - E)^2/E]$, we use OpenOffice Calc CHIDIST to find the corresponding probability from the χ^2 distribution. Just as with the t distribution, we must enter the degrees of freedom. To ascertain these requires some care.

When a comparison is made between one sample and another, as in Table 8.1, a simple rule is that the degrees of freedom equal (number of columns minus one) × (number of rows minus one) (not counting the row and column containing the totals). For the data in Table 8.1, this gives $(2 - 1) \times (5 - 1) = 4$. Another way of looking at this is to ask for the minimum number of figures that must be supplied in Table 8.1, *in addition* to all the totals, to allow us to complete the whole table. Four numbers disposed anyhow in samples A and B, provided they are in separate rows, will suffice.

Using OpenOffice Calc CHIDIST, we find that the probability associated with an X^2 value of 7.147 is 0.13. This is well above the conventionally significant level of 0.05, or 5%, so the null hypothesis *is not* disproved. It is therefore quite conceivable that in the distribution of the patients between socioeconomic classes, the population from which sample A was drawn were the same as the population from which sample B was drawn.

Fourfold tables

A special form of the χ^2 test is particularly common in practice and quick to calculate. It is applicable when the results of an investigation can be set out in a "fourfold table" or "2×2 contingency table".

Consider the isoniazid trial described Table 3.2. For convenience the results are reproduced in Table 8.3.

The null hypothesis is set up that there is no difference between placebo and isoniazid. Using the above method we find $X^2 = 3.418$ and $P = 0.064$. So, despite an apparently considerable difference between the proportions of deaths in the placebo and isoniazid groups, the probability of this result or one more extreme occurring by chance is more than 5%.

We now calculate a confidence interval of the differences between the two proportions, as described in Chapter 5. We could calculate the confidence interval on either the rows or the columns, and it is important that we compare proportions of the outcome variable, that is, death.

$$P_1 = 21/131 = 0.160, \quad P_2 = 11/132 = 0.083, \quad P_1 - P_2 = 0.077$$

$$\mathrm{SE}(P_1 - P_2) = \sqrt{\left(\frac{0.160 \times 0.840}{131} + \frac{0.083 \times 0.917}{132} \right)} = 0.040$$

The 95% confidence interval is:

$$0.077 - 1.96 \times 0.040 \text{ to } 0.077 + 1.96 \times 0.040$$

$$= -0.0014 \text{ to } 0.1555$$

Table 8.3 Results from the isoniazid trial after 6 months follow-up.

	Dead	Alive	Total
Placebo	21	110	131
Isoniazid	11	121	132

Thus the 95% confidence interval is wide, and includes zero, as one might expect because the χ^2 test was not significant at the 5% level.

Small numbers: Yates' correction and Fisher's exact test

When the numbers in a 2×2 contingency table are small, the χ^2 approximation becomes poor. The following recommendations may be regarded as a sound guide.[2] In fourfold tables a χ^2 test is inappropriate if the total of the table is less than 20, or if the total lies between 20 and 40 and the smallest expected (not observed) value is less than 5; in contingency tables with more than one degree of freedom, it is inappropriate if more than about one-fifth of the cells have expected values less than 5 or any cell an expected value of less than 1.

When the values in a fourfold table are fairly small, a "correction for continuity", known as the "Yates' correction", may be applied.[3] Although there is no precise rule defining the circumstances in which to use Yates' correction, a common practice is to incorporate it into χ^2 calculations on tables with a total of under 100 or with any cell containing a value less than 10.

An alternative which is valid for any sample size is known as Fisher's exact test. This is a test which computes the probability of the observed table, given the marginal totals. The one-sided P-value is the sum of the probability of the observed table and tables that yield a smaller probability. A two-sided P-value can be either double the one-sided value or the sum of the probabilities less than the observed one but in the opposite direction. It is "conservative", which means that in general, when the null hypothesis is true it rejects the null hypothesis with a lower probability than we would expect from the preset the type I error rate. To counter this, a mid-P version was introduced, which computes half the value of the observed table and the sum of the more extreme probabilities. This is to be preferred. These are described in detail in earlier versions of this book and all these tests are now routinely available in OpenEpi and OpenStat, and so not discussed further here.

Comparing proportions

Earlier in this chapter we compared two samples by the χ^2 test to answer the question "Are the distributions of the members of these

Table 8.4 People who did or did not get influenza after inoculation with one of five vaccines.

Types of vaccine	Numbers of employees			
	Got influenza	Avoided influenza	Total	Proportion got influenza
I	43	237	280	0.18
II	52	198	250	0.21
III	25	245	270	0.09
IV	48	212	260	0.18
V	57	233	290	0.20
Total	225	1125	1350	

two samples between five classes significantly different?" Another way of putting this is to ask "Are the relative proportions of the two samples the same in each class?"

For example, an industrial medical officer of a large factory wants to immunize the employees against influenza. Five vaccines of various types based on the current viruses are available, but nobody knows which is preferable. From the work force, 1350 employees agree to be immunized with one of the vaccines in the first week of December, so the medical officer randomizes individuals into five approximately equal treatment groups using a computer generated random number scheme. In the first week of the following March, he examines the records he has been keeping to see how many employees got influenza and how many did not. These records are classified by the type of vaccine used (Table 8.4).

In Table 8.4 the figures are analyzed by the χ^2 test. For this we have to determine the expected values. The null hypothesis is that there is no difference between vaccines in their efficacy against influenza. We therefore assume that the proportion of employees contracting influenza is the same for each vaccine as it is for all combined. This proportion is derived from the total who got influenza, and is 225/1350. To find the expected number in each vaccine group who would contract the disease, we multiply the actual numbers in the total column of Table 8.4 by this proportion. Thus $280 \times (225/1350) = 46.7$; $250 \times (225/1350) = 41.7$; and so on. Likewise the proportion who did not get influenza is 1125/1350.

The expected numbers of those who would avoid the disease are calculated in the same way from the totals in Table 8.4, so that

Table 8.5 Calculation of χ^2 test on figures in Table 8.4.

Types of vaccine	Expected numbers		$O - E$		$(O - E)^2/E$	
	Got influenza	Avoided influenza	Got influenza	Avoided influenza	Got influenza	Avoided influenza
I	46.7	233.3	−3.7	3.7	0.293	0.059
II	41.7	208.3	10.3	−10.3	2.544	0.509
III	45.0	225.0	−20.0	20.0	8.889	1.778
IV	43.3	216.7	4.7	−4.7	0.510	0.102
V	48.3	241.7	8.7	−8.7	1.567	0.313
Total	225.0	1125.0	0	0	13.803	2.761

$X^2 = 16.564$, d.f. = 4, $P = 0.002$.

$280 \times (1125/1350) = 233.3$; $250 \times (1250/1350) = 208.3$; and so on. The procedure is thus the same as shown in Tables 8.1 and 8.2.

The calculations made in Table 8.5 show that the X^2 statistic with four degrees of freedom is 16.564, and so $P = 0.002$. This is a highly significant result. But what does it mean?

Splitting of χ^2

Inspection of Table 8.5 shows that the largest contribution to the total X^2 comes from the figures for vaccine III. They are 8.889 and 1.778, which together equal 10.667. If this figure is subtracted from the total X^2, $16.564 - 10.667 = 5.897$. This gives an approximate figure for X^2 for the remainder of the table with three degrees of freedom (by removing the vaccine III we have reduced the table to four rows and two columns). We then find that $P = 0.117$, a non-significant result. However, this is only a rough approximation. To check it exactly we apply the X^2 test to the figures in Table 8.4 minus the row for vaccine III. In other words, the test is now performed on the figures for vaccines I, II, IV, and V. On these figures $X^2 = 2.983$; d.f. = 3; $P = 0.394$. Thus the probability falls within the same broad limits as obtained by the approximate shortcut given above. We can conclude that the figures for vaccine III are responsible for the highly significant result of the total X^2 of 16.564. Some care is needed because we have chosen one value out of a possible five. A very conservative test, known as the Bonferroni test, is to multiply the P-values obtained by the number of tests performed and conclude significance if the value is still less than a critical value such as 5%. In this case the *P*-value associated with an X^2 value of 10.667 with 1 d.f. using OpenOffice Calc CHIDIST is 0.0011, and since 5×0.0011 is 0.0055 this is still well below the conventional 0.05.

But this is not quite the end of the story. Before concluding from these figures that vaccine III is superior to the others, we ought to carry out a check on other possible explanations for the disparity. The process of randomization in the choice of the persons to receive each of the vaccines should have balanced out any differences between the groups, but some may have remained by chance. The sort of questions worth examining now are: Were the people receiving vaccine III as likely to be exposed to infection as those receiving the other vaccines? Could they have had a higher level of immunity from previous infection? Were they of comparable socioeconomic status? Of similar age on average? Were the sexes comparably distributed? Although some of these characteristics could have been more or less balanced by stratified randomization, it is as well to check that they have in fact been equalized before attributing the numeral discrepancy in the result to the potency of the vaccine.

χ^2 test for trend

Table 8.1 is a 5×2 table, because there are five socioeconomic classes and two samples. Socioeconomic groupings may be thought of as an example of an ordered categorical variable, as there are some outcomes (e.g. mortality) in which it is sensible to state that (say) social class II is between social classes I and III. The χ^2 test described at that stage did not make use of this information; if we had interchanged any of the rows, the value of X^2 would have been exactly the same. Looking at the proportions *p* in Table 8.1, we can see that there is no real ordering by social class in the proportions of self-poisoning; social class V is between social classes I and II. However, in many cases, when the outcome variable is an ordered categorical variable, a more powerful test can be devised which uses this information.

Consider a randomized controlled trial of health promotion in general practice to change people's eating habits.[4] Table 8.6 gives the results from a review at 2 years, to look at the change in the proportion eating poultry.

We give each category a score. Usually we choose a linear score and it is convenient to center it on the middle category (although this does not affect the result. Here we have scored the three categories −1, 0, 1. With "a" being the count in for each outcome category in the intervention column, "n" the number of subjects in each outcome category, and "N" the total number of subjects the χ^2 test for trend is calculated in the following way:

$$E_{xp} = \Sigma ax - \frac{\Sigma a \Sigma nx}{N} \quad \text{and} \quad E_{xx} = \Sigma nx^2 - \frac{(\Sigma nx)^2}{N}$$

then

$$X^2 = E_{xp}^2 / (E_{xx}\overline{pq}) \tag{8.1}$$

which yields

$$X^2 = 19.07^2/(269.54 \times 0.5056 \times 0.4944) = 5.20$$

This has one degree of freedom because the linear scoring means that when one expected value is given all the others can be determined directly, and we find $P = 0.02$. The usual χ^2 test gives a value of $X^2 = 5.51$; d.f. = 2; $P = 0.064$. Thus the more sensitive χ^2 test for trend yields a significant result because the test used more information about the experimental design. The values for the scores are to some extent arbitrary. However, it is usual to choose them equally spaced on either side of zero. Thus if there are four groups the scores would be −3, −1, +1, +3, and for five groups −2, −1, 0, +1, +2. The X^2 statistic is quite robust to other values for the scores provided that they are steadily increasing or steadily decreasing. OpenEpi uses a slightly different method known as the Mantel–Haenszel method but gives similar results (Figure 14.10).

Table 8.6 Change in eating poultry in randomized trial.[4]

	Intervention	Control	Total	Proportion in intervention	Score
	a	b	n	p = a/n	X
Increase	100	78	178	0.56	1
No change	175	173	348	0.50	0
Decrease	42	59	101	0.42	−1
Total	317	310	627	0.51	

Note that this is another way of splitting the overall X^2 statistic. The overall X^2 will always be greater than the X^2 for trend, but because the latter uses only one degree of freedom, it is often associated with a smaller probability. Although one is often counseled not to decide on a statistical test after having looked at the data, it is obviously sensible to look at the proportions to see if they are plausibly monotonic (go steadily up or down) with the ordered variable, especially if the overall χ^2 test is non-significant.

Comparison of an observed and a theoretical distribution

In the cases so far discussed, the observed values in one sample have been compared with the observed values in another. But sometimes we want to compare the observed values in one sample with a theoretical distribution.

For example, a geneticist has a breeding population of mice in his laboratory. Some are entirely white, some have a small patch of brown hairs on the skin, and others have a large patch. According to the genetic theory for the inheritance of these colored patches of hair, the population of mice should include 51.0% entirely white, 40.8% with a small brown patch, and 8.2% with a large brown patch. In fact, among the 784 mice in the laboratory 380 are entirely white, 330 have a small brown patch, and 74 have a large brown patch. Do the proportions differ from those expected?

The data are set out in Table 8.7. The expected numbers are calculated by applying the theoretical proportions to the total, namely 0.510×784, 0.408×784, and 0.082×784. The degrees of

Table 8.7 Calculation of X^2 for comparison between actual distribution and theoretical distribution.

Mice	Observed cases	Theoretical proportions	Expected cases	$O - E$	$(O - E)^2/E$
Entirely white	380	0.510	400	−20	1.0000
Small brown patch	330	0.408	320	10	0.3125
Large brown patch	74	0.082	64	10	1.5625
Total	784	1.000	784	0	2.8750

freedom are calculated from the fact that the only constraint is that the total for the expected cases must equal the total for the observed cases, and so the degrees of freedom are the number of rows minus one. Thereafter the procedure is the same as in previous calculations of X^2. In this case X^2 comes to 2.875. Using OpenOffice Calc CHIDIST with 2 d.f. we find that $P = 0.238$. Consequently the null hypothesis of no difference between the observed distribution and the theoretically expected one is *not* disproved. The data conform to the theory.

Chi-squared test for difference in two counts

The total number of deaths in a town from a particular disease varies from year to year. Suppose that in 1 year we had observed O_1 deaths and in the subsequent year O_2 deaths and we wished to test whether there had been a change between the 2 years (provided our attention had not been drawn to a sudden change). Under a null hypothesis of no change between the 2 years, we would expect $E = (O_1 + O_2)/2$ deaths in each year. Then a chi-squared test of the change would be:

$$X^2 = \frac{(O_1 - E)^2}{E} + \frac{(O_2 - E)^2}{E}$$

It is simple to show that this becomes:

$$X^2 = \frac{(O_1 - O_2)^2}{(O_1 + O_2)} \tag{8.2}$$

It is important to note that the deaths must be independently caused; for example, they must not be the result of an epidemic such as influenza. The reports of the deaths must likewise be independent; for example, the criteria for diagnosis must be consistent from year to year and not suddenly change in accordance with a new fashion or test, and the population at risk must be the same size over the period of study.

In spite of its limitations this method has its uses. For instance, in the town of Carlisle, the number of deaths from ischemic heart disease for 1 year was 276. Is this significantly higher than the total for the previous year, which was 246? The difference is 30. The chi-squared test is $\chi^2 = 30^2/(276 + 246) = 1.72$. Using OpenOffice

Calc CHIDIST with 1 d.f. gives $P = 0.2$. The difference could therefore easily be a chance fluctuation.

This method should be regarded as giving no more than approximate but useful guidance, and is unlikely to be valid over a period
of more than very few years owing to changes in diagnostic techniques. An extension of it to the study of paired alternatives follows.

Paired alternatives

As stated earlier, paired data can arise in crossover trials where a
subject has one treatment followed by another, or in a matched
case–control study, where a case is matched by certain characteristics with a control. Consider the example of paired data as
described in Table 3.9. The significance of the results can then be
simply tested by *McNemar's test*. As discussed in Chapter 3, the pairs
of results where both case and control have an event, or where
both case and control fail to have an event (with numbers e and h,
respectively) can be discarded. Thus *conditional* on observing only
one event, under the null hypothesis of no difference between
cases and controls, the *expected* number of events for both cases and
controls is $(f + g)/2$, with observed values f and g.

McNemar's test is then

$$X^2 = \frac{(f - g)^2}{(f + g)} \quad \text{with 1 d.f.}$$

or with a continuity correction,

$$X_c^2 = \frac{(|f - g| - 1)^2}{f + g} \quad \text{with 1 d.f.}$$

The data from Table 3.11 yield

$$X^2 = \frac{(10 - 23)^2}{(10 + 23)} = 5.12$$

or

$$X_c^2 = \frac{(|10 - 23| - 1)^2}{(10 + 23)} = 4.36$$

We find that for the χ^2 values, each with 1 d.f., $P = 0.024$ and $P = 0.037$, respectively. This calculation is also shown using OpenEpi in Figure 14.11.

Extensions of the χ^2 test

If the outcome variable in a study is nominal, the χ^2 test can be extended to look at the effect of more than one input variable, for example, to allow for confounding variables. This is most easily done using *multiple logistic regression*, a generalization of *multiple regression*, which is described in Chapter 11. If the data are matched, then a further technique (*conditional logistic regression*) should be employed. These are described in more detail in *Statistics at Square Two*.

Common questions

There are a number of tests of association for a 2×2 table. Which should I choose?

When the numbers are large it matters little which test to use. When the numbers are small, one should be cautious in placing too much emphasis on differing results. However in general I prefer the mid-P exact test because it generally has better properties.

I have matched data, but the matching criteria were very weak. Should I use McNemar's test?

The general principle is that if the data are matched in any way, the analysis should take account of it. If the matching is weak, then the matched analysis and the unmatched analysis should agree. In some cases when there are a large number of pairs with the same outcome, it would appear that the McNemar's test is discarding a lot of information, and so is losing power. However, imagine we are trying to decide which of two high jumpers is the better. They each jump over a bar at a fixed height, and then the height is increased. It is only when one fails to jump a given height and the other succeeds that a winner can be announced. It does not matter how many jumps both have cleared.

Formula appreciation

We will see a similar equation to (8.1) in equation (11.2) in the regression chapter, which suggests the chi-squared test for trend is in fact a form of regression and so has similar assumptions, such as linearity. Note that in equation (8.2), we do not need to know the size of the population from which the cases came. This is because it is assumed to be the same from one year to the next, and the expected values can be calculated simply from the observed counts.

Reading and reporting chi-squared tests

- It is convention to use the Greek χ^2 to denote the test and the distribution, but the Latin X^2 for the observed statistic, such as "from the χ^2 test we obtained $X^2 = 5.1...$"
- Chi-squared tests with many degrees of freedom are often ill-specified and the results should be treated with caution. If non-significant, they do not imply that certain results are unlikely by chance, and if significant it is unclear what has been proven.
- Report the X^2 statistic, the degrees of freedom, and the P-values, with the estimated difference and a 95% confidence interval for the true difference. Thus in the isoniazid example, we write $X^2 = 3.418$, d.f. = 1, $P = 0.064$, difference in proportions 0.077, 95% confidence interval -0.0014 to 0.1555.

Exercises

8.1 In a trial of new drug against a standard drug for the treatment of depression, the new drug caused some improvement in 56% of 73 patients and the standard drug some improvement in 41% of 70 patients. The results were assessed in five categories as follows:

New treatment: much improved 18, improved 23, unchanged 15, worse 9, much worse 8; Standard treatment: much improved 12, improved 17, unchanged 19, worse 13, much worse 9.

What is the value of X^2 which takes no account of the ordered value of data, what is the value of the X^2 test for trend, and the P-value? How many degrees of freedom are there? What is the value of P in each case?

8.2 An outbreak of pediculosis capitis is being investigated in a girls' school containing 291 pupils. Of 130 children who live in a nearby housing estate 18 were infested and of 161 who live elsewhere 37 were infested. What is the X^2 value of the difference, and what is its significance? Find the difference in infestation rates and a 95% confidence interval for the difference.

8.3 The 55 affected girls were divided at random into two groups of 29 and 26. The first group received a standard local application and the second group a new local application. The efficacy of each was measured by clearance of the infestation after one application. By this measure the standard application failed in ten cases and the new application in five. What is the X^2 value of the difference (with Yates' correction), and what is its significance? What is the difference in clearance rates and an approximate 95% confidence interval?

8.4 A general practitioner reviewed all patient notes in four practices for 1 year. Newly diagnosed cases of asthma were noted, and whether or not the case was referred to hospital. The following referrals were found (total cases in parentheses): practice A, 14 (103); practice B, 11 (92); practice C, 39 (166); practice D, 31 (221). What are the X^2 and P-values for the distribution of the referrals in these practices? Do they suggest that any one practice has significantly more referrals than others?

8.5 Carry out a chi-squared test on the data from Table 3.4 to determine if there is an association between therapy and death or shunt in the PHVD trial. How does this correspond with the results of the confidence interval calculation in Exercise 5.5?

8.6 Carry out a chi-squared test on the data from Table 3.6 to determine if there is an association between hay fever and eczema. How does this result compare with the results for the confidence intervals for odds ratios in Exercise 5.6?

8.7 Carry out a chi-squared test on the data from Table 5.1 to determine if there is a gender difference in appendicitis rates. Given that the estimate of the log odds ratio is 0.170, and its standard error is 0.203, find the corresponding P-value from the z statistic. Contrast the P-values.

8.8 A dermatologist tested a new topical application for the treatment of psoriasis on 48 patients. He applied it to the lesions on one part of the patient's body and what he considered to be the best traditional remedy to the lesions on another but comparable part of the body, the choice of area being made by the toss of a coin. In three patients both areas of psoriasis responded; in 28 patients the disease responded to the traditional remedy but hardly or not at all to the new one; in 13 it responded to the new one but hardly or not at all to the traditional remedy; and in four cases neither remedy caused an appreciable response. Did either remedy cause a significantly better response than the other?

Note in this exercise the purpose of the study would be to determine which treatment to try first, in the absence of any further information. Clearly, if the first treatment fails, there is little lost in trying the other.

References

1. Snedecor GW and Cochran WG. *Statistical Methods*, 7th ed. Iowa: Iowa State University Press, 1980:47.
2. Cochran WG. Some methods for strengthening the common χ^2 tests. *Biometrics* 1956;**10**:417–51.
3. Yates F. Contingency tables involving small numbers and the χ^2 test. *J Roy Stat Soc* Suppl 1934;**1**:217–3.
4. Cupples ME and McKnight A. Randomised controlled trial of health promotions in general practice for patients at high cardiovascular risk. *BMJ* 1994;**309**:993–6.

CHAPTER 9
Diagnostic tests

To consider the evaluation of a diagnostic test, we have to suppose initially that there is a definite way to decide if someone has a particular condition. For example, to diagnose a cancer, one could take a biopsy, to diagnose depression one could conduct an interview with a psychiatrist, and to diagnose a walking problem one could video a patient and have it viewed by an expert. This is sometimes called the "gold standard" (since currencies used to be valued against gold). Often the gold standard test is expensive and difficult to administer. We require a test which is cheaper and easier to use. Initially we will consider a simple binary situation in which both the gold standard and the diagnostic test have either a positive or negative outcome (disease is present or absent).

The situation is best summarized by the ubiquitous 2×2 Table 9.1. In writing this table, always put the gold standard on the top and the results of the test on the side.

Table 9.1 Standard table for diagnostic tests.

		Gold standard		
		Positive	Negative	
Diagnostic test	Positive	a	b	$a + b$
	Negative	c	d	$c + d$
	Total	$a + c$	$b + d$	$n = a + b + c + d$

Statistics at Square One, XIth edition. By M.J. Campbell and T.D.V. Swinscow. Published 2009 by Blackwell Publishing, ISBN: 9781405191005.

The numbers "*a*" and "*d*" are the numbers of true positives and negatives, respectively. The number "*b*" is the number of false positives, because although the test is positive the subjects don't have the disease, and similarly "*c*" is the number of false negatives.

Example:
Consider the study by Kroenke *et al.*[1] who surveyed 965 people attending primary care centers in the USA. They were interested in whether a family practitioner can diagnose generalized anxiety disorder (GAD). They asked two simple questions (the GAD2 questionnaire): "Over the last 2 weeks, how often have you been bothered by the following problems?" (1) feeling nervous, anxious, or on edge and (2) not able to stop or control worrying. The patients answered each question from "not at all", "several days", "more than half the time", and "nearly every day", scoring from 0, 1, 2, 3, respectively. The scores for the two questions were summed and a score of over 3 was considered positive. Two mental health professionals then held structured psychiatric interviews with the subject over the telephone to diagnose GAD. The professionals were ignorant of the result of the GAD2 questionnaire.

The results from Kroenke *et al.*'s study are given in Table 9.2.

We now want to derive some summary statistics from these tables. These are the *prevalence*, the *sensitivity*, and *specificity* of the test, and the *positive predictive value (PPV)*.

The *prevalence* of the disease is the proportion of people diagnosed by the gold standard and is given by $(a + c)/n$. For the GAD example it is $73/965 = 0.076 = 7.6\%$.

Given a person has the disease, the *sensitivity* of the test is the proportion of people who have a positive result on the diagnostic test. This is given by $a/(a + c) = 63/73 = 0.86$.

Table 9.2 Results from Kroenke *et al.*[1]

		Diagnosis by mental health professional		
		Positive	Negative	
GAD2	≥3 (+ve)	63	152	215
	<3 (−ve)	10	740	750
	Total	73	892	965

Suppose a test is 100% sensitive. Then the number of false negatives is zero and we would expect Table 9.3.

Now suppose a patient has a negative test result. From Table 9.3 we can see this means we can be certain that the patient *does not* have the disease. Sackett *et al.* (1997) refer to this as SnNout, that is for a test with a high sensitivity (Sn), a negative result rules *out* the disease.

Given a person does not have the disease, the *specificity* of the test is the proportion of people who have a negative result on the diagnostic test. This is given by $d/(b + d)$. For the GAD example it is $740/892 = 83\%$.

Suppose a test is 100% specific. Then the number of false positives is zero and we would expect Table 9.4.

Now suppose a patient has a positive test result. From Table 9.4, we can see this means we can be certain the patient *has* the disease. Sackett *et al.*[2] refer to this as SpPin., that is for a test with a high specificity (Sp), a positive test rules *in* the disease.

Useful mnemonic

SeNsitivity = 1 − proportion false negatives (*n* in each side)

SPecificity = 1 − proportion false positives (*p* in each side)

What subjects really want to know, however, is "if I have a positive test, what are the chances I have the disease?" This is given by

Table 9.3 Results of a diagnostic test with 100% sensitivity.

		Gold standard		
		Positive	Negative	
Diagnostic test	Positive	a	b	a + b
	Negative	0	d	d
	Total	a	b + d	

Table 9.4 Results of a diagnostic test with 100% specificity.

		Gold standard		
		Positive	Negative	
Diagnostic test	Positive	a	0	a
	Negative	c	d	c + d
	Total	a + c	d	n

the Positive Predictive Value (PPV) which is $a/(a+b)$. For the GAD example this is $63/215 = 29\%$. The probability of an event given a negative predictive test is $c/(c + d) = 1.3\%$. One way of looking at the test is that before the test the chances of having GAD were 7.6%. After the test they are either 29% or 1.3% depending on the result, but note that even with a positive test the chances of having GAD are only about 1/3.

Sensitivity and specificity are independent of prevalence; positive predictive value is not

To show this suppose that in a different population the prevalence of the disease is double that of the current population (assume the prevalence is low, so that a and c are much smaller than b and d and so the results for those without the disease are much the same as the earlier table). The situation is given in Table 9.5.

We see that the sensitivity is now $2a/(2a + 2c) = a/(a + c)$ as before. The specificity is unchanged. However, the PPV is given by $2a/(2a + b)$ which is greater than the earlier value of $a/(a + b)$ (if a is very small relative to b, then the PPV increases directly as the prevalence increases). This highlights that sensitivity and specificity are characteristics of the *test* and will be valid for different populations with different prevalences. Thus we could use them in populations with high prevalence, such as elderly people, as well as with low prevalence, such as for young people. However, the PPV is a characteristic of the *population* and so will vary depending on the prevalence. In general, where the prevalence is low, even a positive result will mean it is likely that one has the disease, as will be shown in Exercise 9.1.

Table 9.5 Standard situation but with a doubling of the prevalence.

		Gold standard		
		Positive	Negative	
Diagnostic test	Positive	$2a$	b	$2a + b$
	Negative	$2c$	d	$2c + d$
	Total	$2a + 2c$	$b + d$	

Likelihood ratio

It is common to prefer a single summary measure, and for a diagnostic test the most useful measure is the likelihood ratio for a positive test LR(+). This is defined as:

$$LR(+) = \frac{\text{Probability of positive test given the disease}}{\text{Probability of positive test without disease}}$$

$$= \frac{\text{Sensitivity}}{1 - \text{specificity}}$$

For the GAD example we find that LR(+) = 0.86/(1 − 0.83) = 5.06.

One reason why this is useful is that we can use it to calculate the odds of having the disease given a positive result. Recall from Chapter 3 that the odds of an event are defined as $p/(1 - p)$, where p is the probability of the event. Before the test is conducted, the probability of having the disease is just the prevalence, and the odds are simply $\{(a + c)/n\}/\{b + d)/n\} = (a + c)/(b + d)$. Thus for GAD, the odds are 0.082 which are close to the prevalence of 0.076 because the prevalence is quite low.

A useful result is derived from what is known as Bayes' theorem and states:

Odds of disease after positive test = odds of disease before
 test × LR(+)

We can get the odds after a positive test directly from the PPV since the odds of disease after a positive test is PPV/(1 − PPV). For the GAD example odds = 0.29/(1 − 0.29) = 0.41.

We can also get this from Bayes' theorem since:

Odds of disease before test × LR(+) = 0.082 × 5.06 = 0.41

Thus knowing the LR(+) gives a simple way to estimate how likely someone is to have a disease, if one knows the prevalence or probability of disease before the test, without having to set up the 2×2 table.

It is important to recall that the sensitivity, specificity, and LR(+) are all *estimates*. They have an associated uncertainty attached to them, and methods of estimating this are discussed in Chapter 5. OpenEpi, as a matter of course, gives confidence intervals for these values as shown in Chapter 14.

ROC curves

For a diagnostic test that produces results on a continuous or ordinal scale, we need to select a convenient cut-off value to calculate the sensitivity and specificity. For example, the GAD2 questionnaire has possible values from 0 to 6. Why should one choose the value of 3 as the cut-off? For a cut-off of 2 the sensitivity is 0.95, the specificity is 0.64, and the LR(+) is 2.6.[1] One might argue that since a cut-off of 3 has a better LR(+) then one should use it. However, a cut-off of 2 gives a higher sensitivity, which might be important. It should be noted that a sensitivity of 100% is always achievable by stating that everyone has the disease, but this is at the expense of a poor specificity (similarly a 100% specificity can be achieved by stating no one has the disease. If the prevalence is low, this tactic will have a high accuracy, that is it will be right most of the time, but sadly wrong for the important cases). A discussion of the different scenarios for preferring a high specificity or sensitivity is given in the next section. A simple graphical device for displaying the trade-offs between sensitivity and specificity is a *receiver operating characteristics* (ROC) curve (the unusual name originates from electrical engineering). This is a plot of sensitivity versus one minus specificity for different cut-off values. A putative plot for the diagnosis of anxiety by different cut-offs on the GAD2 questionnaire is shown in Figure 9.1. The line of equality is also shown, which is what one would expect if the test had no power to detect disease.

ROC curves are particularly useful for comparing different diagnostic plots, a plot which is consistently nearer the left-hand side and the top is to be preferred. However, further consideration is beyond this book and the reader is referred to Machin and Campbell[3] (Chapter 10).

Diagnosis and screening

There is an important distinction between diagnosing a disease and screening for it. In the former case, there are usually some symptoms, and so we already suspect that the patient has something wrong with them. If a test is positive we will take some action. In the latter case, there are usually no symptoms, and so if the test is negative the person will have no further tests. Recalling Sackett's mnemonics SpPin and SnNout, for diagnosis we want a positive test to rule people in, so we want a high specificity. For screening

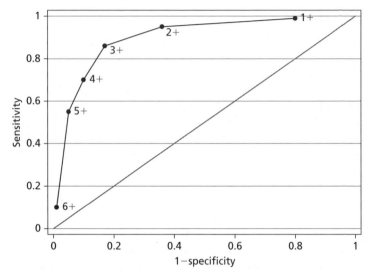

Figure 9.1 An ROC curve for different cut-offs on the GAD2 questionnaire (Kroenke *et al.*[1]) showing the different cut-off values and the line of equality.

we want a negative test to rule people out, so we want a high sensitivity. Thus mass mammography will have a fairly low threshold of suspicion, to ensure a high sensitivity and reduce the chances of missing someone with breast cancer. The subsequent biopsy of positive results will have a high specificity to ensure that if, say, mastectomy is to be considered, the doctor is pretty sure that the patient has breast cancer.

As a final point, it is worth mentioning that there are a number of conditions to be met before one would instigate a mass screening program. One is that catching the disease early makes a difference to prognosis. Another is that there is a treatment available if we did diagnose a patient with a disease. Based on the paper by Kroenke *et al.*, should GPs begin screening for anxiety? The answer in general is no; in the absence of trials showing improved patient benefit and the lack of simple treatments for generalized anxiety, it would be difficult to justify screening an asymptomatic population.

Reading and reporting diagnostic tests

1 Always report confidence intervals measures of sensitivity and specificity.
2 Always report the prevalence of the condition, or if reading a paper, check that it is reported since this will change one's interpretation of the predictive value.
3 Report how the subjects were chosen for the diagnostic test.
4 Question whether treatment would be changed depending on the result of a diagnostic test.

Exercises

9.1 The prevalence of a disease is 1 in 1000. A test has a sensitivity of 100% and specificity of 95%. What is the probability a person has the disease given a positive result on the test? (Hint, think of a population with 10 000 people.)

9.2 Suppose the prevalence of diabetes is 3%. A urine test has a likelihood ratio for a positive test of 15. What is the probability that a person with a positive test has diabetes?
(a) 0.31; (b) 0.45; or (c) 0.98.

9.3 The following statements are true or false:
(a) Sensitivity depends on prevalence. (b) The ROC curve is a graph of sensitivity versus specificity. (c) Specificity is one minus the proportion of false positives. (d) For a screening test we require a high specificity.

References

1. Kroenke K, Spitzer RL, Williams JB, Monahan PO and Löwe B. Anxiety disorders in primary care: prevalence, impairment, comorbidity and detection. *Ann Intern Med* 2007;**146**:317–25.
2. Sackett DL, Richardson WS, Rosenberg W and Haynes RB. *Evidence Based Medicine*. Churchill Livingstone, 1997;102
3. Machin D and Campbell MJ. *Design of Studies for Medical Research*. Chichester: John Wiley and Sons Ltd, 2005.

CHAPTER 10

Rank score tests

Population distributions are characterized, or defined, by parameters such as the mean and standard deviation. For skew distributions, we would need to know other parameters such as the degree of skewness before the distribution could be identified uniquely, but the mean and standard deviation identify the Normal distribution uniquely. The *t* test described earlier depends for its validity on an assumption that the data originate from a Normally distributed population, and, when two groups are compared, the difference between the two samples arises simply because they differ only in their mean value. However, if we were concerned that the data did not originate from a Normally distributed population, then there are tests available which do not make use of this assumption. Because the data are no longer Normally distributed, the distribution cannot be characterized by a few parameters, and so the tests are often called "non-parametric". This is somewhat of a misnomer because, as we shall see, to be able to say anything useful about the population we must compare parameters. As was mentioned in Chapter 6, if the sample sizes in both groups are large, lack of Normality is of less concern, and the large sample tests described in that chapter would apply.

The author Wilcoxon and the authors Mann and Whitney separately described rank sum tests, which have since been shown to be the same. Convention has now ascribed the Wilcoxon test to paired data and the Mann–Whitney *U* test to unpaired data.

Paired samples

Boogert *et al.*[1] (data also given in Shott[2]) used ultrasound to record fetal movements before and after chorionic villus sampling. The

Statistics at Square One, XIth edition. By M.J. Campbell and T.D.V. Swinscow.
Published 2009 by Blackwell Publishing, ISBN: 9781405191005.

Table 10.1 Wilcoxon test on fetal movement before and after chorionic villus sampling.[1,2]

Patient number	Before sampling (2)	After sampling (3)	Difference (before–after) (4)	Rank (5)	Signed rank (6)
1	25	18	7	9	9
2	24	27	−3	5.5	−5.5
3	28	25	3	5.5	5.5
4	15	20	−5	8	−8
5	20	17	3	5.5	5.5
6	23	24	−1	1.5	−1.5
7	21	24	−3	5.5	−5.5
8	20	22	−2	3	−3
9	20	19	1	1.5	1.5
10	27	19	8	10	10

percentage of time the fetus spent moving is given in Table 10.1 for 10 pregnant women.

If we are concerned that the differences in percentage of time spent moving are unlikely to be Normally distributed we could use the Wilcoxon signed rank test using the following assumptions:

1 The paired differences are independent.

2 The differences come from a symmetrical distribution.

We do not need to perform a test to ensure that the differences come from a symmetrical distribution: an "eyeball" test will suffice. A plot of the differences in column (4) of Table 10.1 is given in Figure 10.1 and shows that distribution of the differences is plausibly symmetrical. The differences are then ranked in column (5) (negative values are ignored and zero values omitted). When two or more differences are identical, each is allotted the point half way between the ranks they would fill if distinct, irrespective of the plus or minus sign. For instance, the differences of −1 (patient 6) and +1 (patient 9) fill ranks 1 and 2. As $(1 + 2)/2 = 1.5$, they are allotted rank 1.5. In column (6) the ranks are repeated for column (5), but to each is attached the sign of the difference from column (4). A useful check is that the sum of the ranks must add to $n(n + 1)/2$. In this case $10(10 + 1)/2 = 55$.

The numbers representing the positive ranks and the negative ranks in column (6) are added up separately and only the smaller

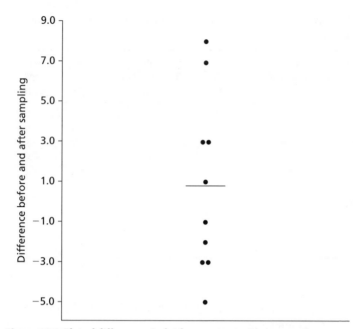

Figure 10.1 Plot of differences in fetal movement with mean value.

of the two totals is used. In this case the smaller of the ranks is 23.5. For $n > 10$ we calculate:

$$z = \frac{|T - n(n+1)/4|}{\sqrt{n(n+1)(2n+1)/24}}$$

On the null hypothesis that the difference in pairs has a mean of zero, z is approximately Normally distributed with mean zero and standard deviation one.

From the data of Table 10.1 we find that:

$$z = \frac{|23.5 - 10 \times 11/4|}{\sqrt{10 \times 11 \times 21/24}} = 0.408$$

From Table A (Appendix) we find P to be about 0.69.

For values of n less that 10, there are tables available from www.faculty.vasser.edu/lowry.

Let T be the smaller of the ranks and let n be the number of pairs. A confidence interval associated with the test is described by Campbell and Gardner[3] and Altman *et al.*,[4] and is easily obtained from the program CIA[5] or from an R program described in Chapter 14. The median difference is zero. CIA gives the 95% confidence interval as -2.50 to 4.00. This is quite narrow and so from this small study we can conclude that we have little evidence that chorionic villus sampling alters the movement of the fetus.

Note, perhaps contrary to intuition, that the Wilcoxon test, although a rank test, may give a different value if the data are transformed, say by taking logarithms. Thus it may be worth plotting the distribution of the differences for a number of transformations to see if they make the distribution appear more symmetrical.

Unpaired samples

A senior registrar in the rheumatology clinic of a district hospital has designed a clinical trial of a new drug for rheumatoid arthritis.

Twenty patients were randomized into two groups of 10 to receive either the standard therapy A or a new treatment B. The plasma globulin fractions after treatment are listed in Table 10.2.

We wish to test whether the new treatment has changed the plasma globulin, and we are worried about the assumption of Normality.

The first step is to plot the data (Figure 10.2).

The clinician was concerned about the lack of Normality of the underlying distribution of the data and so decided to use a non-parametric test. The appropriate test is the Mann–Whitney U test and is computed as follows.

The observations in the two samples are combined into a single series and ranked in order, but in the ranking the figures from one sample must be distinguished from those of the other. The data appear as set out in Table 10.3. To save space they have been set out in two columns, but a single ranking is done. The figures for sample B are set in bold type. Again the sum of the ranks is $n(n + 1)/2$.

Table 10.2 Plasma globulin fraction after randomization to treatment A or B.

Treatment A	38	26	29	41	36	31	32	30	35	33
Treatment B	45	28	27	38	40	42	39	39	34	45

The ranks for the two samples are now added separately, and the smaller total is used. Let n_1 = number of patients or objects in the smaller sample and T_1 the total of the ranks for that sample. If there are only a few ties, that is if two or more values in

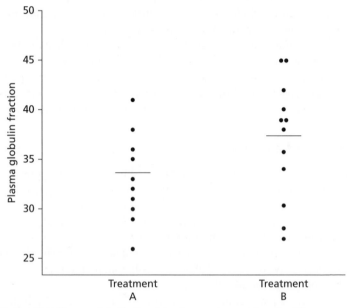

Figure 10.2 Plasma globulin fraction after treatments A or B with mean values.

Table 10.3 Combined results of Table 10.2 (Group B in bold).

Globulin fraction	Rank	Globulin fraction	Rank
26	1	36	11
27	2	38	12.5
28	3	**38**	12.5
29	4	**39**	14.5
30	5	**39**	14.5
31	6	**40**	16
32	7	41	17
33	8	**42**	18
34	9	**45**	19.5
35	10	**45**	19.5

the data are equal (say less than 10% of the data) then we can calculate:

$$z = \frac{|T_1 - n_1(n_1 + n_2 + 1)/2|}{\sqrt{[n_1 n_2 (n_1 + n_2 + 1)/12]}}$$

On the null hypothesis that the two samples come from the same population, z is approximately Normally distributed, mean zero, and standard deviation one, and can be referred to Table A (Appendix) to calculate the P-value.

From the data of Table 10.2 we obtain:

Totals of ranks: sample A, 81.5; sample B, 128.5.

$$z = \frac{|81.5 - 10 \times 21/2|}{\sqrt{(10 \times 10 \times 21/12)}} = 1.78$$

and from Table A (Appendix) we find that P is about 0.075. Again for smaller sample sizes, tables are available at www.faculty.vasser.edu/lowry/.

To calculate a meaningful confidence interval, we assume that if the two samples come from different populations the distribution of these populations differs only in that one appears shifted to the left or right of the other. This means, for example, that we do not expect one sample to be strongly right skewed and one to be strongly left skewed. If the assumption is reasonable, then a confidence interval for the median difference can be calculated.[3,4] Note that the computer program does not calculate the difference in medians, but rather the median of all possible differences between the two samples. This is usually close to the median difference and has theoretical advantages. From CIA we find that the difference in medians is −5.5 and the approximate 95% confidence interval is −10 to 1.0 and similar values are found using R (Table 14.14b). As might be expected from the significance test, this interval includes zero. Although this result is not significant, it would be unwise to conclude that there was no evidence that treatments A and B differed because the confidence interval is quite wide. This suggests that a larger study should be planned.

Non-Normally distributed data can sometimes be transformed by the use of logarithms or some other method to make them Normally distributed, and a t test performed. Consequently the best procedure to adopt may require careful thought. The extent and nature of the difference between two samples is often brought out more clearly by standard deviations and t tests than by non-parametric tests.

It is an interesting observation that the Mann–Whitney U test is unaffected by simple transformations, but the Wilcoxon signed rank test is affected. This is because the rank of a set of numbers and rank of (say) the log of these numbers are the same. However, the rank of the *difference* in a set of numbers and the rank of the difference in their logs are not necessarily the same.

Both the Wilcoxon and Mann–Whitney U test can be carried out using OpenStat (Chapter 14), but at the time of writing it does not give confidence intervals.

Common questions

Non-parametric tests are valid for both non-Normally distributed data and Normally distributed data, so why not use them all the time?

It would seem prudent to use non-parametric tests in all cases, which would save one the bother of testing for Normality. Parametric tests are preferred, however, for the following reasons:

1 As I have tried to emphasize in this book, we are rarely interested in a significance test alone; we would like to say something about the population from which the samples came, and this is best done with estimates of parameters and confidence intervals.

2 It is difficult to do flexible modeling with non-parametric tests, for example allowing for confounding factors using multiple regression (see Chapter 11).

Do non-parametric tests compare medians?

It is a commonly held belief that a Mann–Whitney U test is in fact a test for differences in medians. However, two groups could have the same median and yet have a significant Mann–Whitney U test. Consider the following data for two groups, each with 100 observations. Group 1: 98 (0), 1, 2; Group 2: 51 (0), 1, 48 (2). The median in both cases is 0, but from the Mann–Whitney test $P < 0.0001$.

Only if we are prepared to make the additional assumption that the difference in the two groups is simply a shift in location (i.e. the distribution of the data in one group is simply shifted by a fixed amount from the other) can we say that the test is a test of the difference in medians. However, if the groups have the same distribution, then a shift in location will move medians and means by the same amount and so the difference in medians is the same as the difference in means. Thus the Mann–Whitney U test is also a test for the difference in means.

How is the Mann–Whitney *U* test related to the *t* test?

If one were to input the ranks of the data rather than the data themselves into a two sample t test program, the P-value obtained would be very close to that produced by a Mann–Whitney U test.

Reading and reporting rank score tests

When reading a result from a non-parametric test, one is often faced with a bald P-value. One should then ask what hypothesis is being tested? As shown above, one has to make further assumption before statements concerning parameters such as means can be made.

A Mann–Whitney U test such as that described earlier should be reported as "Mann–Whitney $P = 0.075$, difference in medians -5.5, 95% CI -10 to 1.0". Often, because of inappropriate software, confidence intervals for non-parametric tests are not reported, but there are now a number of packages which will calculate them. For the two sample test, a confidence interval is only interpretable if the distribution of the outcome is similar in the two groups; if the distributions are markedly different, then the two groups differ in more than just a shift in location. Differences in spread can be as important as differences in medians.[6]

Exercises

10.1 A new treatment in the form of tablets for the prophylaxis of migraine has been introduced, to be taken before an impending attack. Twelve patients agree to try this remedy in addition to the usual general measures they take, subject to advice from their doctor on the taking of analgesics also. A crossover trial with identical placebo tablets is carried out over a period of 8 months. The numbers of attacks experienced by each patient on, first, the new treatment and, secondly, the placebo were as follows: patient (1) 4 and 2; patient (2) 12 and 6; patient (3) 6 and 6; patient (4) 3 and 5;

patient (5) 15 and 9; patient (6) 10 and 11; patient (7) 2 and 4; patient (8) 5 and 6; patient (9) 11 and 3; patient (10) 4 and 7; patient (11) 6 and 0; patient (12) 2 and 5. In a Wilcoxon rank sum test, what is the smaller total of ranks? Is it significant at the 5% level?

10.2 Another doctor carried out a similar pilot study with this preparation on 12 patients, giving the same placebo to 10 other patients. The numbers of migraine attacks experienced by the patients over a period of 6 months were as follows.

Group receiving new preparation: patient (1) 8; (2) 6; (3) 0; (4) 3; (5) 14; (6) 5; (7) 11; (8) 2
Group receiving placebo: patient (9) 7; (10) 10; (11) 4; (12) 11; (13) 2; (14) 8; (15) 8; (16) 6; (17) 1; (18) 5.

In a Mann–Whitney two sample test, what is the smaller total of ranks? Which sample of patients provides it? Is the difference significant at the 5% level?

References

1. Boogert A, Manhigh A and Visser GHA. The immediate effects of chorionic villus sampling on fetal movements. *Am J Obstet Gynecol* 1987;**157**:137–9.
2. Shott S. *Statistics for Health Professionals*. Philadelphia: WB Saunders, 1990.
3. Campbell MJ and Gardner MJ. Calculating confidence intervals for some non-parametric analyses. *BMJ* 1988;**296**:1369–71.
4. Altman DG, Machin D, Bryant T and Gardner MJ. *Statistics with Confidence. Confidence Intervals and Statistical Guidelines*, 2nd ed. London: BMJ Publishing Group, 2000:37–9.
5. Bryant TN. *CIA (Confidence Interval Analysis)*. London: BMJ Publishing Group, 2000.
6. Hart A. Mann–Whitney test is not just a test of medians: differences in spread can be important. *BMJ* 2001:**323**:391–3.

CHAPTER 11

Correlation and regression

The word *correlation* is used in everyday life to denote some form of association. We might say that we have noticed a correlation between foggy days and attacks of wheeziness. However, in statistical terms, we use correlation to denote association between two quantitative variables. We also assume that the association is *linear*, that one variable increases or decreases a fixed amount for a unit increase or decrease in the other. The other technique that is often used in these circumstances is *regression*, which involves estimating the best straight line to summarize the association.

Correlation coefficient

The degree of association is measured by a correlation coefficient, denoted by *r*. It is sometimes called Pearson's correlation coefficient after its originator and is a measure of linear association. If a curved line is needed to express the relationship, other and more complicated measures of the correlation must be used.

The correlation coefficient is measured on a scale that varies from +1 through 0 to −1. Complete correlation between two variables is expressed by either +1 or −1. When one variable increases as the other increases the correlation is positive; when one decreases as the other increases it is negative. Complete absence of correlation is represented by 0. Figure 11.1 gives some graphical representations of correlation.

Looking at data: scatter diagrams

When an investigator has collected two series of observations and wishes to see whether there is a relationship between them, he

Statistics at Square One, XIth edition. By M.J. Campbell and T.D.V. Swinscow.
Published 2009 by Blackwell Publishing, ISBN: 9781405191005.

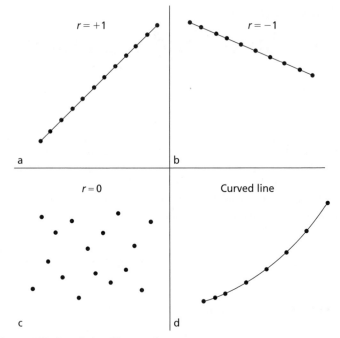

Figure 11.1 Correlation illustrated.

or she should first construct a scatter diagram. The vertical scale represents one set of measurements and the horizontal scale the other. If one set of observations consists of experimental results and the other consists of a time scale or observed classification of some kind, it is usual to put the experimental results on the vertical axis. These represent what is called the "dependent variable". The "independent variable", such as time or height or some other observed classification, is measured along the horizontal axis, or baseline.

The words "independent" and "dependent" could puzzle the beginner because it is sometimes not clear what is dependent on what. This confusion is a triumph of common sense over misleading terminology, because often each variable is dependent on some third variable, which may or may not be mentioned. It is reasonable, for instance, to think of the height of children as dependent on age rather than the converse, but consider a positive correlation between mean tar yield and nicotine yield of certain brands of cigarette[1]. The nicotine liberated is unlikely to have its origin in the tar: both vary in parallel with some other factor or factors in the composition of the cigarettes. The yield of the one does not seem to be "dependent" on the other in the sense that, on average, the height of a child depends on his age. In such cases, it often does not matter which scale is put on which axis of the scatter diagram. However, if the intention is to make inferences about one variable from the other, the observations *from which* the inferences are to be made are usually put on the baseline. As a further example, a plot of monthly deaths from heart disease against monthly sales of ice cream would show a negative association. However, it is hardly likely that eating ice cream protects from heart disease! It is simply that the mortality rate from heart disease is inversely related—and ice cream consumption is positively related—to a third factor, namely environmental temperature.

Calculation of the correlation coefficient

A pediatric registrar has measured the pulmonary anatomical dead space (in ml) and height (in cm) of 15 children. The data are given in Table 11.1 and the scatter diagram is shown in Figure 11.2. Each dot represents one child, and it is placed at the point corresponding to the measurement of the height (horizontal axis) and the dead space (vertical axis). The registrar now inspects the pattern to see whether it seems likely that the area covered by the dots centers on a straight line or whether a curved line is needed. In this case, the pediatrician decides that a straight line can adequately describe the general trend of the dots. His next step will therefore be to calculate the correlation coefficient.

When making the scatter diagram (Figure 11.2) to show the heights and pulmonary anatomical dead spaces in the 15 children, the pediatrician set out figures as in Columns (1), (2), and (3) of Table 11.1. It is helpful to arrange the observations in serial order of the independent variable when one of the two variables is clearly identifiable as independent. The corresponding figures for the dependent variable can then be examined in relation to the increasing series for the independent variable. In this way, we get the same picture, but in numerical form, as it appears in the scatter diagram.

The calculation of the correlation coefficient is as follows, with x representing the values of the independent variable (in this case

Table 11.1 Height and pulmonary anatomical dead space in 15 children.

Child number (1)	Height (cm) (2)	Dead space (ml), y (3)
1	110	44
2	116	31
3	124	43
4	129	45
5	131	56
6	138	79
7	142	57
8	150	56
9	153	58
10	155	92
11	156	78
12	159	64
13	164	88
14	168	112
15	174	101
Total	2169	1004
Mean	144.6	66.933

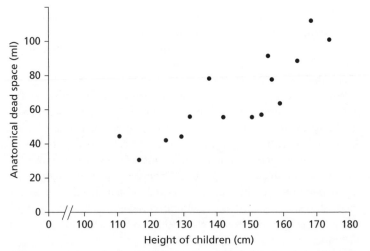

Figure 11.2 Scatter diagram of relation in 15 children between height and pulmonary anatomical dead space.

height) and y representing the values of the dependent variable (in this case anatomical dead space). The formula to be used is:

$$r = \frac{\Sigma(x - \bar{x})(y - \bar{y})}{\sqrt{\left[\Sigma(x - \bar{x})^2\Sigma(y - \bar{y})^2\right]}} \qquad (11.1)$$

Using OpenStat as shown in Chapter 14, we find that:

$$r = 0.846$$

If we wish to label the strength of the association, for absolute values of r, 0–0.19 is regarded as very weak, 0.2–0.39 as weak, 0.40–0.59 as moderate, 0.6–0.79 as strong, and 0.8–1 as very strong correlation, but these are rather arbitrary limits, and the context of the results should be considered. The correlation coefficient of 0.846 indicates a very strong positive correlation between size of pulmonary anatomical dead space and height of child. But in interpreting correlation, it is important to remember that *correlation is not causation*. There may or may not be a causative connection between the two correlated variables. Moreover, if there *is* a connection it may be indirect.

A part of the variation in one of the variables (as measured by its variance) can be thought of as being due to its relationship with the other variable and another part as due to undetermined (often "random") causes. The part due to the dependence of one variable on the other is measured by r^2. For these data, $r^2 = 0.716$ so we can say that 72% of the variation between children in size of the anatomical dead space is accounted for by the height of the child.

Significance test

To test whether the association is merely apparent, and might have arisen by chance, use the t test in the following calculation:

$$t = r\sqrt{\frac{n - 2}{1 - r^2}} \qquad (11.2)$$

where t has $n - 2$ degrees of freedom.

For example, the correlation coefficient for these data was 0.846. The number of pairs of observations was 15. Applying equation (11.2), we have:

$$t = 0.846 \sqrt{\frac{15 - 2}{1 - 0.846^2}} = 5.72.$$

Using OpenOffice Calc TDIST with $15 - 2 = 13$ degrees of freedom, we find that $P < 0.001$ so the correlation coefficient may be regarded as highly significant. Thus (as could be seen immediately from the scatterplot), we have a very strong correlation between dead space and height which is most unlikely to have arisen by chance.

The assumptions governing this test are:
- that both variables are plausibly Normally distributed;
- that there is a linear relationship between them;
- the null hypothesis is that there is no association between them.

The test should not be used for comparing two methods of measuring the same quantity, such as two methods of measuring peak expiratory flow rate. Its use in this way appears to be a common mistake, with a significant result being interpreted as meaning that one method is equivalent to the other. The reasons have been extensively discussed,[2] but it is worth recalling that a significant result tells us little about the strength of a relationship.

Spearman rank correlation

A plot of the data may reveal outlying points well away from the main body of the data, which could unduly influence the calculation of the correlation coefficient. Alternatively, the variables may be quantitative discrete such as a mole count, or ordered categorical such as a pain score. A non-parametric procedure, due to Spearman, is to replace the observations by their ranks in the calculation of the correlation coefficient.

This results in a simple formula for the Spearman rank correlation, r_s.

$$r_s = 1 - \frac{6\Sigma d^2}{n(n^2 - 1)}$$

where d is the difference in the ranks of the two variables for a given individual. Thus we can derive Table 11.2 from the data in Table 11.1.

Table 11.2 Derivation of Spearman's rank correlation from data of Table 11.1.

Child number	Rank height	Rank dead space	d	d²
1	1	3	2	4
2	2	1	−1	1
3	3	2	−1	1
4	4	4	0	0
5	5	5.5	0.5	0.25
6	6	11	5	25
7	7	7	0	0
8	8	5.5	−2.5	6.25
9	9	8	−1	1
10	10	13	3	9
11	11	10	−1	1
12	12	9	−3	9
13	13	12	−1	1
14	14	15	1	1
15	15	14	−1	1
Total				60.5

From this we get that:

$$r_s = 1 - \frac{6 \times 60.5}{15 \times (225 - 1)} = 0.8920$$

In this case the value is very close to that of the Pearson correlation coefficient. For $n > 10$, the Spearman rank correlation coefficient can be tested for significance using the t test given earlier.

The regression equation

Correlation describes the strength of an association between two variables, and is completely symmetrical, the correlation between A and B is the same as the correlation between B and A. However, if the two variables are related, it means that when one changes by a certain amount the other changes on an average by a certain amount. For instance, in the children described earlier greater height is associated, on average, with greater anatomical dead space. If y represents the dependent variable and x the independent variable, this relationship is described as the regression of y on x.

The relationship can be represented by a simple equation called the *regression equation*. In this context "regression" (the term is a historical anomaly) simply means that the average value of *y* is a "function" of *x*, that is, it changes with *x*.

The regression equation representing how much *y* changes with any given change of *x* can be used to construct a *regression line* on a scatter diagram, and in the simplest case this is assumed to be a straight line. The direction in which the line slopes depends on whether the correlation is positive or negative. When the two sets of observations increase or decrease together (positive), the line slopes upwards from left to right; when one set decreases as the other increases, the line slopes downwards from left to right. As the line must be straight, it will probably pass through few, if any, of the dots. Given that the association is well described by a straight line, we have to define two features of the line if we are to place it correctly on the diagram. The first of these is its distance above the baseline; the second is its slope. They are expressed in the following *regression equation*:

$$y = \alpha + \beta x$$

With this equation we can find a series of values of y_{fit}, the variable, that correspond to each of a series of values of *x*, the independent variable. The parameters α and β have to be estimated from the data. The parameter α signifies the distance above the baseline at which the regression line cuts the vertical (*y*) axis; that is, when $x = 0$. The parameter β (the *regression coefficient*) signifies the amount by which change in *x* must be multiplied to give the corresponding average change in *y*, or the amount *y* changes for a unit increase in *x*. In this way, it represents the degree to which the line slopes upwards or downwards.

The regression equation is often more useful than the correlation coefficient. It enables us to predict *y* from *x* and gives us a better summary of the relationship between the two variables. If, for a particular value of *x*, x_i, the regression equation predicts a value of y_{fit}, the prediction error is $y_i - y_{\text{fit}}$. It can easily be shown that *any* straight line passing through the mean values $\bar{x}$ and $\bar{y}$ will give a total prediction error $\Sigma(y_i - y_{\text{fit}})$ of zero because the positive and negative terms exactly cancel. To remove the negative signs, we square the differences and the regression equation chosen to minimize the sum of squares of the prediction errors, $S^2 = \Sigma(y_i - y_{\text{fit}})^2$ We denote the sample estimates of α and β by *a* and *b*. It can be shown that the one straight line that minimizes S^2, the *least squares estimate*, is given by:

$$b = \frac{\Sigma(x - \bar{x})(y - \bar{y})}{\Sigma(x - \bar{x})^2} \qquad (11.3)$$

and

$$a = \bar{y} - b\bar{x}$$

Using OpenStat as shown in Chapter 14, we find $b = 1.033$ ml/cm and $a = -82.4$ ml.

Therefore, in this case, the equation for the regression of y on x becomes:

$$y = -82.4 + 1.033x$$

This means that, on average, for every increase in height of 1 cm, the increase in anatomical dead space is 1.033 ml *over the range of measurements made*.

The line representing the equation is shown superimposed on the scatter diagram of the data in Figure 11.3.

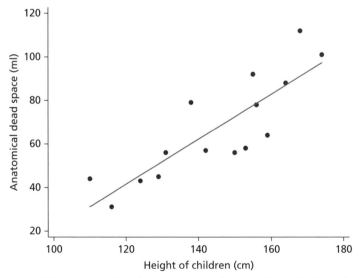

Figure 11.3 Regression line drawn on scatter diagram relating height and pulmonary anatomical dead space in 15 children (Table 11.2).

The standard error of the slope SE(b) is given by:

$$SE(b) = \frac{S_{res}}{\sqrt{\Sigma(x - \bar{x})^2}} \qquad (11.4)$$

where S_{res} is the residual standard deviation, given by:

$$S_{res} = \sqrt{\frac{\Sigma(y - y_{fit})^2}{n - 2}}$$

We find SE(b) = 13.08445/72.4680 = 0.18055.

We can test whether the slope is significantly different from zero by:

$$t = b/SE(b) = 1.033/0.18055 = 5.72$$

Again, this has $n - 2 = 15 - 2 = 13$ degrees of freedom. The assumptions governing this test are:

- That the *prediction errors* are approximately Normally distributed. Note this does not mean that the x or y variables have to be Normally distributed.
- That the relationship between the two variables is linear.
- That the scatter of points about the line is approximately constant—we would not wish the variability of the dependent variable to be growing as the independent variable increases. If this is the case, try taking logarithms of both the x and y variables.

Note that the test of significance for the slope gives exactly the same value of P as the test of significance for the correlation coefficient. Although the two tests are derived differently, they are algebraically equivalent, which makes intuitive sense, since a test for a significant correlation should be the same as a test for a significant slope.

We can obtain a 95% confidence interval for b from

$$b - t_{0.05} \times SE(b) \text{ to } b + t_{0.05} \times SE(b)$$

where the t statistic has 13 degrees of freedom, and from OpenOffice Calc TINV is found to be 2.160.

Thus the 95% confidence interval is:

$$1.033 - 2.160 \times 0.18055 \text{ to } 1.033 + 2.160 \times 0.18055$$

$$= 0.643 \text{ to } 1.422.$$

Regression lines give us useful information about the data they are collected from. They show how one variable changes on average with another, and they can be used to find out what one variable is likely to be when we know the other—provided that we ask this question within the limits of the scatter diagram. To project the line at either end—to extrapolate—is always risky because the relationship between x and y may change or some kind of cut-off point may exist. For instance, a regression line might be drawn relating the chronological age of some children to their bone age, and it might be a straight line between, say, the ages of 5 and 10 years, but to project it up to the age of 30 would clearly lead to error. Computer packages will often produce the intercept from a regression equation, with no warning that it may be totally meaningless. Consider a regression of blood pressure against age in middle aged men. The regression coefficient is often positive, indicating that blood pressure increases with age. The intercept is often close to zero, but it would be wrong to conclude that this is a reliable estimate of the blood pressure in newly born male infants!

More advanced methods

More than one independent variable is possible—in such a case the method is known as *multiple regression*. This is the most versatile of statistical methods and can be used in many situations. Examples include: to allow for more than one predictor, age as well as height in the above example; to allow for covariates—in a clinical trial the dependent variable may be outcome after treatment, the first independent variable can be binary, 0 for placebo, and 1 for active treatment, and the second independent variable may be a baseline variable, measured before treatment, but likely to affect outcome. Further details are given in *Statistics at Square Two.*

Common questions

If two variables are correlated are they causally related?

It is a common error to confuse correlation and causation. All that correlation shows is that the two variables are associated. There may be a third variable, a *confounding* variable that is related to both of them. For example, as stated earlier, monthly deaths by drowning and monthly sales of ice cream are positively correlated, but no one would say the relationship was causal!

How do I test the assumptions underlying linear regression?

Firstly always look at the scatterplot and ask, is it linear? If the relationship is plausibly linear, fit the regression equation and calculate the residuals $e_i = y_i - y_{fit}$. A histogram of e_i will reveal departures from Normality. A plot of e_i versus y_{fit} will reveal whether the residuals increase in size as y_{fit} increases and if this is the case then the assumption about a constant variance is unlikely to be true.

When should I use correlation and when should I use regression?

If there is a clear causal pathway, then generally it is better to use regression, although quoting the correlation coefficient as a measure of the strength of the relationship is helpful. In epidemiological surveys, where one is interested only in the *strength* of a relationship, then correlations are preferable. For example, in a survey comparing ovarian cancer rates by country, with the sales of oral contraceptives, it is the existence of a relationship that is of interest, and so a correlation coefficient would be a useful summary.

Which are the important assumptions for linear regression?

The most important assumption is that the relationship is linear. The slope can be vulnerable to "outliers" which are points well away from the main body of data. The next most important assumption is that the observations are independent and especial care is needed when the data for a time series.

What is the relationship between regression and the *t* test?

In the two sample *t* test example, suppose we entered the transit times as a single column, which we call *y*, with one group followed by the second, we also entered a second column with 1 = Treatment A and 2 = Treatment B, which we call *x*. Then the *p*-value associated with the regression of *y* on *x* is the same as that for the *t* test comparing Treatments A and B, and the regression coefficient is the contrast between A and B, (mean(B)–mean(A)) with a 95% confidence interval.

Formula appreciation

One can see that if one swaps x and y in equation (11.1) the outcome stays the same. Thus for a correlation coefficient it does not matter which variable is the dependent one and which the independent one. Also in equation (11.1), if we put $y = x$ we get $r = 1$ and if we put $y = -x$ we get $r = -1$. From the formula (11.2), it should be clear that even with a very weak relationship (say $r = 0.1$), we would get a significant result with a large enough sample (say n over 1000). Formula (11.3) contrasts with formula (11.1) since now the result *will* change if one swaps x and y. Formula (11.4) shows that one can achieve a small standard error by having a wide range of x, so that the denominator is large. What this means in practice is that if one was investigating a relationship, for example the relationship between lung volume and height, it would be sensible to collect data on some very short people and some very tall people!

Reading and reporting correlation and regression

- Make clear what type of correlation coefficient is being used (e.g. Pearson or Spearman).
- Ask whether the relationship is really linear. Do the authors produce evidence that the model is reasonable? For example, do they discuss the distribution of the residuals?
- Quote the correlation coefficient and its P-value, or the regression slope, 95% confidence interval for the slope, the t statistic, degrees of freedom, and P-value. Thus for the data from Table 11.1, we would write, "regression slope of dead space against height is 1.033 ml/cm (95% CI 0.643 to 1.422), $P < 0.001$, $r = 0.846$.

Exercises

11.1 A study was carried out into the attendance rate at a hospital of people in 16 different geographical areas over a fixed period of time. The distance of the center from the hospital of each area was measured in miles. The results were as follows:

(1) 21%, 6.8; (2) 12%, 10.3; (3) 30%, 1.7; (4) 8%, 14.2; (5) 10%, 8.8; (6) 26%, 5.8; (7) 42%, 2.1; (8) 31%, 3.3; (9) 21%, 4.3; (10) 15%, 9.0; (11) 19%, 3.2; (12) 6%, 12.7; (13) 18%, 8.2; (14) 12%, 7.0; (15) 23%, 5.1; (16) 34%, 4.1.

Plot the data. Is the relation plausibly linear? What is the correlation coefficient between the attendance rate and mean distance of the geographical area?

11.2 Find the Spearman rank correlation for the data given in Exercise 11.1.

11.3 In Exercise 11.1, let x represents mean distance of the area from the hospital and y represents attendance rates. What is the equation for the regression of y on x? What does it mean?

11.4 Find the standard error and 95% confidence interval for the slope of the data in Exercise 11.1.

11.5 Playing with the data. If the results for area 12 in question 11.1 were 6%, 22.7, how does this change the correlation coefficient, the Spearman's rank correlation, and the regression slope. If the results for area 6 were 10%, 5.8, how would that affect the results?

References

1. Russell MAH, Cole PY, Idle MS and Adams L. Carbon monoxide yields of cigarettes and their relation to nicotine yield and type of filter. *BMJ* 1975;**3**:71–3.

2. Bland JM and Altman DG. Statistical methods for assessing agreement between two methods of clinical measurement. *Lancet* 1986;**i**:307–10.

CHAPTER 12

Survival analysis

Survival analysis is concerned with studying the time between entry to a study and a subsequent event. Originally the analysis was concerned with time from treatment until death, hence the name, but survival analysis is applicable to many areas as well as mortality. Recent examples include time to discontinuation of a contraceptive, maximum dose of bronchoconstrictor required to reduce a patient's lung function to 80% of baseline, time taken to exercise to maximum tolerance, time that a transdermal patch can be left in place, time for a leg fracture to heal.

When the outcome of a study is the time between one event and another, a number of problems can occur.

- The times are most unlikely to be Normally distributed.
- We cannot afford to wait until events have happened to all the subjects, for example until all are dead. Thus some patients will still be alive at the close of the study. Other patients might have left the study early—they are *lost to follow up*. Thus the only information we have about some patients is that they were still alive until some point in time. These are termed *censored observations*.

Kaplan–Meier survival curve

We look at the data using a Kaplan–Meier survival curve.[1] Suppose that the survival times, including censored observations, after entry into the study (ordered by increasing duration) of a group of

Statistics at Square One, XIth edition. By M.J. Campbell and T.D.V. Swinscow.
Published 2009 by Blackwell Publishing, ISBN: 9781405191005.

n subjects are t_1, t_2,...t_n. The proportion of subjects, $S(t)$, surviving beyond any follow-up time (t_p) is estimated by:

$$S(t) = \frac{(r_1 - d_1)}{r_1} \times \frac{(r_2 - d_2)}{r_2} \cdots \times \cdots \frac{r_p - d_p}{r_p}$$

where t_p is the largest survival time less than or equal to t and r_i is the number of subjects alive just before time t_i (the ith ordered survival time), d_i denotes the number who died at time t_i where i can be any value between 1 and p. For censored observations $d_i = 0$.

Method

Order the survival time by increasing duration starting with the shortest one. At each event (i) work out the number alive immediately before the event (r_i). Before the first event all the patients are alive and so $S(t) = 1$. If we denote the start of the study as t_o, where $t_0 = 0$, then we have $S(t_0) = 1$. We can now calculate the survival times t_i, for each value of i from 1 to n by means of the following recurrence formula.

Given the number of events (deaths), d_i, at time t_i and the number alive, r_i, just before t_i calculate

$$S(t_i) = \frac{r_i - d_i}{r_i} \times S(t_{i-1})$$

We do this only for the events and not for censored observations. The survival curve is unchanged at the time of a censored observation, but at the next event after the censored observation the number of people "at risk" is reduced by the number censored between the two events.

Example of calculation of survival curve

McIllmurray and Turkie[2] describe a clinical trial of 49 patients for the treatment of Dukes' C colorectal cancer. The data for the two treatments, γ linolenic acid or control are given in Table 12.1.[2,3]

The calculation of the Kaplan–Meier survival curve for the 25 patients randomly assigned to receive γ linolenic acid is described in Table 12.2. The + sign indicates censored data. Until 6 months after treatment, there are no deaths, so $S(t) = 1$. The effect of the censoring is to remove from the alive group those that are censored.

Table 12.1 Survival in 49 patients with Dukes' C colorectal cancer randomly assigned to either γ linolenic acid or control treatment.

Treatment	Survival time (months)
γ Linolenic acid ($n = 25$)	1+, 5+, 6, 6, 9+, 10, 10, 10+, 12, 12, 12, 12, 12+, 13+, 15+, 16+, 20+, 24, 24+, 27+, 32, 34+, 36+, 36+, 44+
Control ($n = 24$)	3+, 6, 6, 6, 6, 8, 8, 12, 12, 12+, 15+, 16+, 18+, 18+, 20, 22+, 24, 28+, 28+, 28+, 30, 30+, 33+, 42

Table 12.2 Calculation of survival case for 25 patients randomly assigned to receive γ linolenic acid.

Case (i)	Survival time (months) (t_i)	Number alive (r_i)	Deaths (d_i)	Proportion surviving $(r_i - d_i)/r_i$	Cumulative proportion surviving $S(t)$
	0	0	0	–	1
1	1+	25	0	1	1
2	5+	24	0	1	1
3	6	23	2	0.9130	0.9130
4	6				
5	9+	21	0	1	0.9130
6	10	20	2	0.90	0.8217
7	10				
8	10+				
9	12	17	4	0.7647	0.6284
10	12				
11	12				
12	12				
13	12+				
14	13+	12	0	1	0.6284
15	15+	11	0	1	0.6284
16	16+	10	0	1	0.6284
17	20+	9	0	1	0.6284
18	24	8	1	0.875	0.5498
19	24+				
20	27+	6	0	1	0.5498
21	32	5	1	0.80	0.4399
22	34+				
23	36+				
24	36+				
25	44+				

At time 6 months two subjects have been censored and so the number alive just before 6 months is 23. There are two deaths at 6 months.

Thus,

$$S(6) = \frac{1 \times (23 - 2)}{23} = 0.9130$$

We now reduce the number alive ("at risk") by two. The censored event at 9 months reduces the "at risk" set to 20. At 10 months there are two deaths, so the proportion surviving is $18/20 = 0.90$ and the cumulative proportion surviving is $0.913 \times 0.90 = 0.8217$. As one can see, the effect of the censored observations is to reduce the number at risk without affecting the survival curve $S(t)$. The survival curve is shown in Figure 12.1. The censored observations are shown as ticks on the line.

Finally we plot the survival curve, as shown in Figure 12.1. The censored observations are shown as ticks on the line.

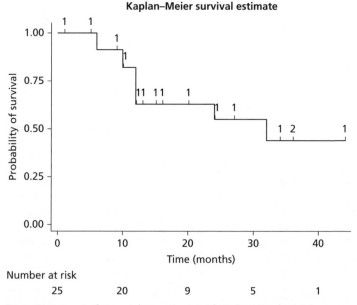

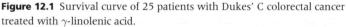

Figure 12.1 Survival curve of 25 patients with Dukes' C colorectal cancer treated with γ-linolenic acid.

Log rank test

To compare two survival curves produced from two groups A and B, we use the rather curiously named log rank test,[1] so called because it can be shown to be related to a test that uses the logarithms of the ranks of the data.

The assumptions used in this test are:

- That the survival times are ordinal or continuous.
- That the risk of an event in one group relative to the other does not change with time. Thus if linolenic acid reduces the risk of death in patients with colorectal cancer, then this risk reduction does not change with time (the so-called *proportional hazards assumption*).

We first order the data for the two groups combined, as shown in Table 12.3. As for the Kaplan–Meier survival curve, we now consider each event in turn, starting at time $t = 0$.

At each event (death) at time t_i we consider the total number alive (r_i) and the total number still alive in group A (r_{Ai}) up to that point. If we had a total of d_i events at time t_i, then, under the null

Table 12.3 Calculation of log rank statistics for 49 patients randomly assigned to receive γ linolenic acid (A) or control (B).

Survival time months (t_i)	Group	Total at risk (r)	Number of events (d_i)	Total at risk in group A (r_{Ai})	Expected number of events in A (E_{Ai})
0		49			
1+	A	49	0	25	0
3+	B	48	0	24	0
5+	A	47	0	24	0
6	A	46	6	23	3.0
6	A				
6	B				
6	B				
6	B				
6	B				
8	B	40	2	21	1.05
8	B				
9+	A	38	0	21	0

Continued

Table 12.3 Continued

Survival time months (t_i)	Group	Total at risk (r)	Number of events (d_i)	Total at risk in group A (r_{Ai})	Expected number of events in A (E_{Ai})
10	A	37	2	20	1.0811
10	A				
10+	A				
12	A	34	6	17	3.0
12	A				
12	A				
12	A				
12	B				
12	B				
12+	A				
12+	B				
13+	A	26	0	12	0
15+	A	25	0	11	0
15+	B	24	0	10	0
16+	A	23	0	10	0
16+	B	22	0	9	0
18+	B	21	0	9	0
18+	B				
20	B	19	1	9	0.4736
20+	A				
22+	B	17	0	8	0
24	A	16	2	8	1.0
24	B				
24+	A				
27+	A	13	0	6	0
28+	B	12	0	5	0
28+	B				
28+	B				
30	B	9	1	5	0.5555
30+	B				
32	A	7	1	5	0.7143
33+	B	6	0	4	0
34+	A	5	0	4	0
36+	A	4	0	3	0
36+	A				
42	B	2	1	1	0.50
44+	A				

hypothesis, we consider what proportion of these would have been expected in group A. Clearly the more people at risk in one group the more deaths (under the null hypothesis) we would expect.

Thus the number of events in group A is:

$$E_{Ai} = \frac{r_{Ai}}{r_i} \times d_i$$

The effect of the censored observations is to reduce the numbers at risk, but they do not contribute to the expected numbers.

Finally, we add the total number of expected events in group A,

$$E_A = \Sigma E_{Ai}$$

If the total number of events in group B is E_B, we can deduce E_B from $E_B = n - E_A$, where n is the total number of events. We do not calculate the expected number beyond the last event, in this case at time 42 months. Also, we would stop calculating the expected values if any survival times greater than the point we were at were found in one group only.

Finally, to test the null hypothesis of equal risk in the two groups, we compute:

$$X^2 = \frac{(O_A - E_A)^2}{E_A} + \frac{(O_B - E_B)^2}{E_B}$$

where O_A and O_B are the total number of events in groups A and B. We compare X^2 to a χ^2 distribution with one degree of freedom (one, because we have two groups and one constraint, namely that the total expected events must equal the total observed).

The calculation for the colorectal data is given in Table 12.3. The first non-censored event occurs at 6 months, at which there are six events. By that time 46 patients are at risk, of whom 23 are in group A. Thus we would expect $6 \times 23/46 = 3$ to be in group A. At 8 months we have $46 - 6 = 40$ patients at risk of whom $23 - 2 = 21$ are in group A. There are two events, of which we would expect $2 \times 21/40 = 1.05$ to occur in group A.

The total expected number of events in A is $E_A = 11.3745$. The total number of events is 22, $O_A = 10$, $O_B = 12$. Thus $E_B = 10.6255$.

Thus

$$X^2 = \frac{(10 - 11.37)^2}{11.37} + \frac{(12 - 10.63)^2}{10.63} = 0.34$$

We compare this with the χ^2 table using OpenCalc CHIDIST with one degree of freedom to find $P = 0.56$.

The relative risk can be estimated by $r = (O_A/E_A)/(O_B/E_B)$. The standard error of the log risk is given by:[4]

$$\text{SE}(\log(r)) = \sqrt{(1/E_A + 1/E_B)}$$

Thus we find $r = 0.779$ and so $\log(r) = -0.250$, $\text{SE}(\log(r)) = 0.427$, and so an approximate 95% confidence interval for $\log(r)$ is:

$$-1.087 \text{ to } 0.587$$

and so a 95% confidence interval for r is $e^{-1.087}$ to $e^{0.587}$, which is:

$$0.34 \text{ to } 1.80$$

This would imply that γ linolenic acid reduced mortality to about 78% compared with the control group, but with a very wide confidence interval. In view of the very small χ^2 statistic, we have little evidence that this result would not have arisen by chance.

It is simple to obtain the Kaplan–Meier plot and carry out the log rank test using OpenStat as described in Chapter 14.

Further methods

In the same way that multiple regression is an extension of linear regression, an extension of the log rank test is called Cox regression. This models the instantaneous risk at any point in time, known as the hazard and is often known as proportional hazards regression. It was developed by DR Cox and can allow for prognostic factors. It is beyond the scope of this book, but is described in *Statistics at Square Two* and elsewhere.[4]

Common questions

Do I need to test for a constant relative risk before doing the log rank test?

This is a similar problem to testing for Normality for a t test. The log rank test is quite "robust" against departures from proportional hazards, but care should be taken. If the Kaplan–Meier survival curves cross then this is clear departure from proportional hazards, and the log rank test should not be used. This can happen, for example, in a two drug trial for cancer, if one drug is very toxic initially but produces more long term cures. In this case there is no simple answer to the question "is one drug better than the other?", because the answer depends on the time scale.

If I don't have any censored observations, do I need to use survival analysis?

Not necessarily, you could use a rank test such as the Mann–Whitney U test, but the survival method would yield an estimate of risk, which is often required, and lends itself to a useful way of displaying the data.

Reading and reporting survival analysis

- Beware of reading too much into the right hand part of a Kaplan–Meier plot, unless one has data to show that there is still a reasonably sized sample there, since it may be based on very small numbers. As shown in Figure 12.1, one should print the numbers at risk at intervals along the survival time axis.
- For survival curves with a high proportion of survivors, it is helpful to truncate the y-axis, and not plot acres of white space, or plot the cumulative mortality curve $1 - S(t)$ instead. (Further details of plotting survival data are given in Freeman et al.[5])
- Relative risks are difficult to interpret, and for communication it can be helpful to choose a time (say 2 years for the linolenic acid data) and give the estimated proportions surviving at that point.
- The log rank test should be presented as "X^2(log rank) = 0.34, d.f. = 1, P = 0.56. Estimated relative risk 0.427, 95% confidence interval 0.33 to 1.80".

Exercises

12.1 Twenty patients, 10 of normal weight and 10 severely over-weight underwent an exercise stress test, in which they had to lift a progressively increasing load for up to 12 min, but they were allowed to stop earlier if they could do no more. On two occasions the equipment failed before 12 min. The times (in min) achieved were:

Normal weight: 4, 10, 12*, 2, 8, 12*, 8[†], 6, 9, 12*
Overweight: 7[†], 5, 11, 6, 3, 9, 4, 1, 7, 12*

*Reached end of test; [†]equipment failure. (I am grateful to C Osmond for these data).

(a) What are the observed and expected values?

(b) What is the value of the log rank test to compare these groups?

(c) Playing with the data: What is the effect of changing one of the 12^* to 30^*? $8^\dagger$ to $12^\dagger$? 8 to 120?

12.2 What is the risk of stopping in the normal weight group compared with the overweight group, and a 95% confidence interval?

References

1. Peto R, Pike MC, Armitage P, *et al*. Design and analysis of randomised clinical trials requiring prolonged observation of each patient: II. Analysis and examples. *Br J Cancer* 1977;**35**:1–39.

2. McIllmurray MB and Turkie W. Controlled trial of γ-linolenic acid in Dukes' C colorectal cancer. *BMJ* 1987;**294**:1260, **295**:475.

3. Altman DG, Machin D, Bryant TN and Gardner MJ (Eds). *Statistics with Confidence*, 2nd ed. London: BMJ Publishing Group, 2000: Chapter 9.

4. Machin D, Cheung Y-B and Parmar M. *Survival Analysis: A Practical Approach*. Chichester: Wiley, 2006.

5. Freeman JV, Walters SJ and Campbell MJ. *How to Display Data*. Oxford: Wiley-Blackwell, 2007.

CHAPTER 13

Study design and choosing a statistical test

Design

In many ways the design of a study is more important than the analysis. A badly designed study can never be retrieved, whereas a poorly analyzed one can usually be reanalyzed. Consideration of design is also important because the design of a study will govern how the data are to be analyzed. This chapter can only briefly consider the issues and for more details the reader is referred to Machin and Campbell.[1]

Most medical studies consider an input, which may be a medical intervention or exposure to a potentially toxic compound, and an output, which is some measure of health that the intervention is supposed to affect. The simplest way to categorize studies is with reference to the time sequence in which the input and output are studied.

The most powerful studies are *prospective* studies, and the paradigm for these is the *randomized controlled trial*. In this, subjects with a disease are randomized to one of two (or more) treatments, one of which may be a control treatment. Methods of randomization have been described in Chapter 4. The importance of randomization is that we know in the long run (i.e. with a large number of subjects), treatment groups will be balanced in known and *unknown* prognostic factors. However, with small studies, the chances of imbalance in some important prognostic factors are quite high. Another important feature of randomization is that one cannot predict in advance which treatment a patient will receive. This matters, because knowledge of likely treatment may affect

Statistics at Square One, XIth edition. By M.J. Campbell and T.D.V. Swinscow. Published 2009 by Blackwell Publishing, ISBN: 9781405191005.

whether the subject gets recruited into the trial. It is important that the treatments are *concurrent*—that the active and control treatments occur in the same period of time.

To allow for the therapeutic effect of simply being given treatment, the control may consist of a *placebo*, an inert substance that is physically identical to the active compound. If possible a study should be *double blinded*—neither the investigator nor the subject being aware of what treatment the subject is undergoing. Sometimes it is impossible to blind the subjects, for example when the treatment is some form of health education, but often it is possible to ensure that the people evaluating the outcome are unaware of the treatment and this is known as a single blind trial.

A *parallel group* design is one in which treatment and control are allocated to different individuals. Examples of a parallel group trial are given in Table 7.1, in which different bran preparations have been tested on different individuals, Table 8.5 comparing different vaccines, and Table 8.6 evaluating health promotion. A *matched parallel* design comes about when randomization is between matched pairs, such as in Exercise 8.8, in which randomization was between different parts of a patient's body.

A *crossover* study is one in which two or more treatments are applied sequentially to the same subject. Clearly this type of study can only be considered for chronic conditions, where treatment is not expected to cure the patient and where withdrawal of treatment leads to a return to a baseline level which is relatively stable. The advantages are that each subject then acts as their own control and so fewer subjects may be required. The main disadvantage is that there may be a *carryover* effect in that the action of the second treatment is affected by the first treatment. An example of a crossover trial is given in Table 7.2, in which different dosages of bran are compared within the same individual. Another type of trial is a *sequential* trial, when the outcome is evaluated after each patient or a group of patients, rather than after all the patients have been gathered into the study. It is useful if patient recruitment is slow and the outcome evaluated quickly, such as levels of nausea after an anesthetic. *Cluster* trials are trials where groups of patients, rather than individual patients, are randomized. They may occur in primary care, where general practitioners are randomized to different training packages, or public health where different areas receive different health promotion campaigns. Further details on clinical trials are available in a number of excellent books.[2-5]

One of the major threats to validity of a clinical trial is *compliance* (or the more politically correct *adherence*). Patients are likely to drop out of trials if the treatment is unpleasant, and often fail to take medication as prescribed. It is usual to adopt a pragmatic approach and analyze by *intention to treat*, that is analyze the data by the treatment that the subject was *assigned* to, not the one they actually took. Of course, if the patients have dropped out of a trial, it may be impossible to get measurements from them, unless they can be obtained by proxy, such as whether the subject is alive or dead. The alternative to an intention to treat analysis is to analyze *per protocol* or *on study*. The trouble with this type of analysis is that we no longer have a randomized comparison and so comparisons may be biased. Dropouts should be reported by treatment group. Checklists for writing reports on clinical trials are available.[6,7]

A *quasi-experimental* design is one in which treatment allocation is not random. An example of this is given in Exercise 8.8 comparing two locations for an outbreak of pediculosis capitis. These designs are useful for evaluating interventions which have been introduced without trial evidence. One can compare areas of the country where the intervention has been introduced with other areas where it has not. The difficulty lies in interpretation, in that one cannot be sure whether reasons why some areas have the intervention early are also related to the outcome.

A *cohort* study is one in which subjects, initially disease free, are followed up over a period of time. Some will be exposed to some risk factor, for example cigarette smoking. The outcome may be death and we may be interested in relating the risk factor to a particular cause of death. Clearly, these have to be large, long term studies and tend to be costly to carry out. If records have been kept routinely in the past, then a historical cohort study may be carried out, an example of which is the appendicitis study discussed in Chapter 6. Here, the cohort is all cases of appendicitis admitted over a given period and a sample of the records could be inspected retrospectively. A typical example would be to look at birth weight records and relate birth weight to disease in later life.

These studies differ in essence from retrospective studies, which start with diseased subjects and then examine possible exposure. Such *case–control* studies are commonly undertaken as a preliminary investigation, because they are relatively quick and inexpensive. The comparison of the blood pressure in farmers and printers given in Chapter 4 is an example of a case–control study. It is retrospective because we argued from the blood pressure to the occupation and did not start out with subjects assigned to occupation. There are many confounding factors in case–control studies. For example, does occupational stress cause high blood pressure, or do people prone to high blood pressure choose stressful occupations? A particular problem is *recall bias*, in that the cases, with the disease, are more motivated to recall apparently trivial episodes in the past than controls, who are disease free.

Cross-sectional studies are common and include surveys, laboratory experiments, and studies to examine the prevalence of a disease. Studies validating instruments and questionnaires are also cross-sectional studies. The study of urinary concentration of lead in children described in Chapter 1 and the study of the relationship between height and pulmonary anatomical dead space in Chapter 11 are cross-sectional studies. The main problem of cross-sectional studies is ensuring the sample is representative of the population from which it is taken. Different types of sample are described in Chapter 4.

In general, when one is evaluating interventions, randomized trials are considered the best and most reliable form of evidence. However there are important caveats about this. The subjects in randomized trials are volunteers, and so may not be typical of the sort of patient one meets in practice. They tend to be small and of short duration, so rare side effects may not be picked up. It may not be ethical to conduct a trial, if most clinicians believe in the efficacy of the treatment. However observational studies are themselves vulnerable; a classic example is the evaluation of hormone replacement therapy. This appeared to be beneficial for heart disease, but it was likely that women who were at lower risk of heart disease were more likely to ask for it.

Sample size

One of the most common questions asked of a statistician about design is the number of patients to include. It is an important question, because if a study is too small it will not be able to answer the question posed, and would be a waste of time and money. It could also be deemed unethical because patients may be put at risk with no apparent benefit. However, studies should not be too large because resources would be wasted if fewer patients would have sufficed. The sample size for a continuous outcome depends on four critical quantities: the type I and type II error rates α and β (discussed in Chapter 5), the variability of the data σ^2, and the effect size d. In a trial the effect size is the amount by which we would expect the two treatments to differ, or is the minimum difference that would be clinically worthwhile. For a binary outcome we need to specify α and β, and proportions P_1 and P_2, where P_1 is the expected outcome under the control intervention and $P_1 - P_2$ is the minimum clinical difference which it is worthwhile detecting.

Usually α is fixed at 5% and β is fixed at 20% (or 10%). An intuitive way to think of sample size is to think of the distribution of a series of 95% confidence intervals calculated from random samples of the same size, n, under the alternative hypothesis, as shown in Figure 13.1. As n gets larger the confidence intervals will get narrower. However, by definition, 95% of the (95%) confidence intervals will include the mean of the alternative hypothesis, d. A type II error of 20% means that we would expect 20% of the confidence intervals to include the null hypothesis of zero. Thus one way of thinking of power is the proportion of confidence intervals which would exclude the null hypothesis when the alternative hypothesis is true.

A simple formula for a two group parallel trial with a continuous outcome is that the required sample size per group is given by:

$$n = 16\sigma^2/d^2 \text{ for two-sided } \alpha \text{ of 5\% and } \beta \text{ of 20\%}$$

For example, in a trial to reduce blood pressure, if a clinically worthwhile effect for diastolic blood pressure is 5 mmHg and the between subjects standard deviation is 10 mmHg, we would require $n = 16 \times 100/25 = 64$ patients per group in the study. For binary data this becomes $8\ (P_1(1 - P_1) + P_2(1 - P_2))/(P_1 - P_2)^2$. Thus suppose in the PHVD trial of Chapter 3, the standard therapy resulted in 45% of children requiring a shunt or dying. We wished to reduce this to 35%. In the formula we express the percentages as proportions. Then we would require

$$n = 8 \times (0.45 \times 0.55 + 0.35 \times 0.65)/0.1^2$$
$$= 380 \text{ subjects per group}$$

to have an 80% chance of detecting the specified difference at 5% significance. The sample size goes up as the square of the standard deviation of the data (the variance) and goes down inversely as the square of the effect size. Doubling the effect size reduces the sample size by four—it is much easier to detect large effects!

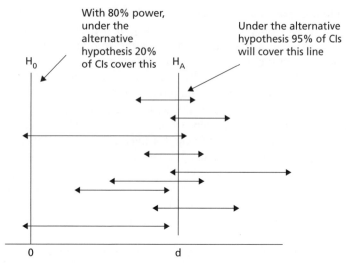

Figure 13.1 Illustration of power using confidence intervals.

In practice, the sample size is often fixed by other criteria, such as finance or resources, and the formula is used to determine a realistic effect size. If this is too large, then the study will have to be abandoned or increased in size. Machin *et al.* give advice on a sample size calculations for a wide variety of study designs.[8] OpenEpi gives sample size and power calculations for a variety of designs for proportions and means.

Choice of test

In terms of selecting a statistical test, the most important question is "what is the main study hypothesis?" In some cases there is no hypothesis; the investigator just wants to "see what is there". For example, in a prevalence study, there is no hypothesis to test, and the size of the study is determined by how accurately the investigator wants to determine the prevalence. If there is no hypothesis, then there is no statistical test. It is important to decide *a priori* which hypotheses are confirmatory (i.e. are testing some presupposed relationship), and which are exploratory (are suggested by the data). No single study can support a whole series of hypotheses.

A sensible plan is to limit severely the number of confirmatory hypotheses. Although it is valid to use statistical tests on hypotheses suggested by the data, the *P*-values should be used only as guidelines, and the results treated as very tentative until confirmed by subsequent studies. A useful guide is to use a *Bonferroni* correction, which states simply that if one is testing *n* independent hypotheses, one should use a significance level of 0.05/*n*. Thus if there were two independent hypotheses, a result would be declared significant only if $P < 0.025$. Note that, since tests are rarely independent, this is a very conservative procedure—one unlikely to reject the null hypothesis.

The investigator should then ask "are the data independent?" This can be difficult to decide but as a rule of thumb results on the same individual, or from matched individuals, are not independent. Thus results from a crossover trial, or from a case–control study in which the controls were matched to the cases by age, sex, and social class, are not independent. It is generally true that the analysis should reflect the design, and so a matched design should be followed by a matched analysis. Results measured over time require special care.[9] One of the most common mistakes in statistical analysis is to treat correlated variables as if they were independent. For example, suppose we were looking at treatment of leg ulcers, in which some people had an ulcer on each leg. We might have 20 subjects with 30 ulcers, but the number of independent pieces of information is 20 because the state of ulcers on each leg for one person may be influenced by the state of health of the person and an analysis that considered ulcers as independent observations would be incorrect. For a correct analysis of mixed paired and unpaired data, consult a statistician.

The next question is "what types of data are being measured?" The test used should be determined by the data. The choice of test for matched or paired data is described in Table 13.1 and for independent data in Figure 13.2.

Table 13.1 Choice of statistical test from paired or matched observation.

Variable	Test
Nominal	McNemar's test
Ordinal (ordered categories)	Wilcoxon
Quantitative (discrete or non-Normal)	Wilcoxon
Quantitative (Normal*)	Paired *t* test

*It is the *difference* between the paired observations that should be plausibly Normal.

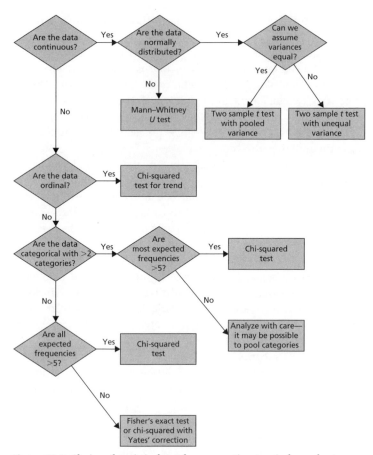

Figure 13.2 Choice of statistical test for comparting two independent groups.

It is helpful to decide the *input* variables and the *outcome* variables. In Figure 13.2 the input variable is binary. For example, in a clinical trial, the input variable is type of treatment—a nominal variable—and the outcome may be some clinical measure, perhaps Normally distributed. The required test is then the *t* test as shown in Figure 13.2. As another example, suppose we have a cross-sectional study in which we ask a random sample of people whether they think their general practitioner is doing a good job, on a five point scale, and we wish to ascertain whether women have a higher opinion of general practitioners than men have. The input variable is gender, which is nominal. The outcome variable is the five point ordinal scale. Each person's opinion is independent of the others, so we have independent data. From Figure 13.1 we should use a χ^2 test for trend, or a Mann–Whitney U test (with correction for ties). Note, however, if some people share a general practitioner and others do not, then the data are not independent and a more sophisticated analysis is called for.

Note that these tables should be considered as guides only, and each case should be considered on its merits. Further help can be obtained from OpenEpi "Intro and Help/choosing a method".

Reading and reporting on the design of a study

- There should always be a succinct statement in the abstract of a report stating the type of study and its size, for example "a case–control study of 50 cases and 60 controls".
- The sample size should be justified by a power-based statement in the methods section. Note that this should be written down *before* the study is carried out. Retrospective power calculations, saying what the power *would* have been, are not helpful; use a confidence interval instead.
- For clinical trials, always report the trial in the manner described by the CONSORT statement[7] (http://www.consort-statement.org/). This includes factors such as how many people were approached to enter the study, how many actually entered, and how many were followed up?

Exercises

State the type of study described in each of the following.

13.1 To investigate the relationship between egg consumption and heart disease, a group of patients admitted to hospital with myocardial infarction were questioned about their egg consumption. A group of age and sex matched patients admitted to a fracture clinic were also questioned about their egg consumption using an identical protocol.

13.2 To investigate the relationship between certain solvents and cancer, all employees at a factory were questioned about their exposure to an industrial solvent, and the amount and length of exposure measured. These subjects were regularly monitored, and after 10 years a copy of the death certificate for all those who had died was obtained.

13.3 A survey was conducted of all nurses employed at a particular hospital. Among other questions, the questionnaire asked about the grade of the nurse and whether she was satisfied with her career prospects.

13.4 To evaluate a new back school, patients with lower back pain were randomly allocated to either the new school or to conventional occupational therapy. After 3 months they were questioned about their back pain, and observed lifting a weight by independent monitors.

13.5 A new triage system has been set up at the local accident and emergency unit. To evaluate it the waiting times of patients were measured for 6 months and compared with the waiting times at a comparable nearby hospital.

References

1. Machin D and Campbell MJ. *The Design of Studies in Medical Research.* Chichester: Wiley, 2006.
2. Pocock SJ. *Clinical trials: A Practical Approach.* Chichester: Wiley, 1983.
3. Senn SJ. *The Design and Analysis of Cross-Over Trials,* 2nd ed. Chichester: Wiley, 2002.
4. Whitehead J. *The Design and Analysis of Sequential Clinical Trials,* revised 2nd ed. Chichester: Wiley, 1997.
5. Donner A and Klar N. *Design and Analysis of Cluster Randomised Trials in Health Research.* London: Arnold, 2000.
6. Gardner MJ, Machin D, Campbell MJ and Altman DG. *Statistical Checklists.* In Altman DG, Machin D, Bryant TN and Gardner MJ (eds), *Statistics with Confidence.* BMJ Publishing Group, 2000.
7. Moher D, Schultz KF and Altman D. The CONSORT Statement: revised recommendations for improving the quality of reports of parallel-group randomized trials. *JAMA* 2001:**285**;1987–91.
8. Machin D, Campbell MJ, Tan SB and Tan SH A. *Statistical Tables for the Design of Clinical Studies,* 3rd ed. Oxford: Wiley-Blackwell, 2009.
9. Matthews JNS, Altman DG, Campbell MJ and Royston JP. Analysis of serial measurements in medical research. *BMJ* 1990;**300**:230–5.

CHAPTER 14
Use of computer software

It is my firmly held view that one has to actually calculate a mean or a relative risk in order to be able to really understand what these concepts mean. Thus in teaching, I feel that students should be able to compute simple statistics using calculators. However, this only needs to be done once and the complexity of the calculations means that rapidly too much time would be taken up in repetitive number crunching. Computers are now ubiquitous and so should be used for more complex calculations. For serious analysis, a commercial package should be used. *Stata* is the package of choice for the more complex statistics used in *Statistics at Square Two*. A proper commercial package will include a spreadsheet database which can handle missing values and category labels. Certain spreadsheets such as Microsoft Excel can also do some statistical analysis, and there are add-ons available to extend their capabilities. A free version of this spreadsheet is *OpenOffice Calc*. It can be used for entering data and performing elementary calculations. It is useful for computing P-values and it enabled me to do away with tables of the chi-squared and t distributions. For example, in *OpenOffice Calc*, given a t-statistic t, and degrees of freedom d.f., and a toggle $m = 1$ for one-sided and $m = 2$ for two-sided tests, to obtain the P-value, all one has to enter in the command line is $= \mathrm{TDIST}(t; \mathrm{d.f.}; m)$. Similarly given probability alpha (two sided), and d.f., to obtain the t-statistic, one has to enter $= \mathrm{TINV}(\mathrm{alpha}; \mathrm{d.f.})$. Similar methods are available for the Normal distribution and the chi-squared distribution.

However, I would not recommend spreadsheets for general statistical analysis. The best and most comprehensive free statistical

Statistics at Square One, XIth edition. By M.J. Campbell and T.D.V. Swinscow.
Published 2009 by Blackwell Publishing, ISBN: 9781405191005.

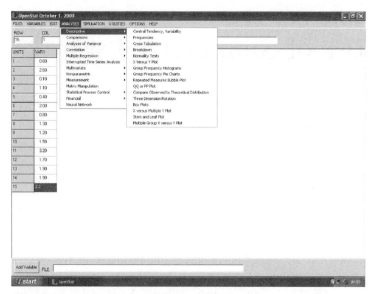

Figure 14.1 *OpenStat* screen showing options for analyzing data from Table 1.2.

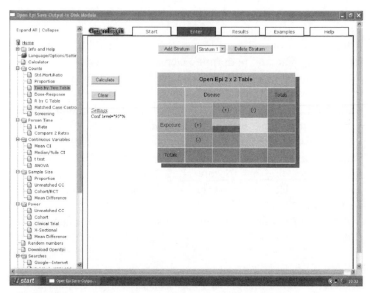

Figure 14.2 Screen dump for *OpenEpi* to analyze a 2×2 table.

package is the *R* package. However, it is not suitable for elementary statistics. A useful, user friendly package that uses *R* programs is *Xycoon*. I have not found a single package that covers all the techniques in this book, but two complementary packages *OpenStat* and *OpenEpi* do cover almost everything. Two other packages, *CHI*, which is home grown, and *SISA* will also do many of the procedures. It is important to appreciate that these are organic packages, and so they are continually being updated, and so the output may not be exactly as it is here. One failure of free software is a decent graphics package (except *R*) and I have used *Stata* to give better figures than I could get from free packages (although the failure might be mine!). Details of the websites are given at the end of the chapter. The packages *OpenEpi*, *SISA*, and *CHI* deal largely with count data, where one can enter the totals directly onto a table on the screen. *OpenStat* has a database and can read data from a large variety of databases or one can enter data directly. One can then cross-tabulate data and carry out analyses such as regression. *OpenStat* also caters for more advanced procedures such as logistic and Cox regression, which are discussed in *Statistics at Square Two*. Figure 14.1 shows a screen dump of *OpenStat*, illustrating procedures for obtaining descriptive statistics for Table1.2. *OpenStat* starts with one variable and one can enter data directly into a column. It is good practice to click the "variables/define" buttons to name the variable and give it a type (floating, integer, string, date, or money) at the start. To add another variable, one clicks the "add variable" button on the bottom left of the screen. Statistical options are available under "analyses", and Figure 14.1 shows what is available under the "descriptive" option.

Figure 14.2 shows a screen dump for *OpenEpi*, illustrating procedures for analyzing a 2×2 table. The options are available on the left hand column.

Chapters 1 and 2: Basic statistics

The stem-and-leaf plot and the box plot are available under "analyses/descriptive" in *OpenStat*. Figure 14.3 shows the results of using the "analyses/descriptive/central tendency, variability" option to obtain the mean and median, the standard deviation, and the interquartile range. As an option, it gives eight other different methods of calculating the quartiles, most of which are the same with this data set. The method given in Chapter 1 which is the default method for *OpenStat* is method 2 in Figure 14.3. Tukey's hinges, described in Chapter 1, is method 5. The*OpenStat* program displays the figures to more accuracy than can be supported by the data and so the results should not be quoted verbatim. Instead, the rules of Chapters 1 and 2 should be applied. The program also gives what are known as the third and fourth moments, namely skewness and kurtosis. Skewness measures the amount of asymmetry in the distribution and kurtosis measures how flat or pointed the distribution is relative to a Normal distribution. Personally I find neither of much use in practical statistics. A simpler measure of skewness is to compare the mean and median, or simply view a histogram of the data.

```
DISTRIBUTION PARAMETER ESTIMATES

================================================================

VAR1 (N = 15)  Sum =         22.500
Mean =      1.500  Variance =       0.711  Std.Dev. =        0.843
Std.Error of Mean =       0.218
 0.950 Confidence Interval for mean :        1.033 to      1.967
Range =       3.100  Minimum =        0.100  Maximum =       3.200
Skewness =        0.220  Std. Error of Skew =       0.580
Kurtosis =       -0.207  Std. Error Kurtosis =       1.121

================================================================

Median =      1.500
Q1 =         0.800
Q3 =         2.000
Interquartile range =       1.200

================================================================

Alternative Methods for Obtaining Quartiles
     Method 1      2        3        4        5        6        7        8
Pcntile
Q1      0.750    0.800    0.800    0.800    0.950    0.800    0.800    0.800
Q2      1.400    1.500    1.500    1.500    1.500    1.500    1.500    1.500
Q3      1.925    2.000    2.000    2.000    1.950    1.900    1.900    2.000
NOTES:
Method 1 is the weighted average at X[np] where n is no. of cases, p
is percentile / 100
Method 2 is the weighted average at X[(n+1)p] This is used in this
program.
Method 3 is the empirical distribution function.
Method 4 is called the empirical distribution function - averaging.
Method 5 is called the empirical distribution function =
Interpolation.
Method 6 is the closest observation method.
Method 7 is from the TrueBasic Statistics Graphics Toolkit.
Method 8 was used in an older Microsoft Excel version.
See the internet site http://www.xycoon.com/ for the above.
```

Figure 14.3 Results of using "analyses/descriptives/central tendency" from OpenStat on data from Table 1.2.

To calculate the mean and standard deviation of grouped data such as in Table 2.2, one needs to weight the outcome by the number of subjects. This can be done in *OpenStat* using the "variables/ create expanded file from frequency data". This then creates a new data set with 140 observations. The frequency variable must have no zeros or decimal places.

Chapter 3

The data from Table 3.2 from a 2×2 table are analyzed in Figure 14.4 using *OpenEpi*'s button "Counts/two by two table". It is important to enter the data in the correct rows, to get the risk ratio in the right direction. The program is mainly intended for epidemiological studies and so for a clinical trial with an intervention and a control, the "exposed" row is the intervention, and the "unexposed" the control. In a clinical trial with two interventions, the "exposed" row would be the new intervention compared with the standard. Thus here "Exposure +" is the isoniazid row and "Exposure −" is the placebo. For "Disease +" we enter the number of deaths and "Disease −" is the number alive. The output corresponds to the results in Chapter 3. The prevented fraction in exposed (pfe) is the same as the relative risk reduction (RRR). The Taylor series method of computing the confidence intervals is the same as that given in the chapter.

Chapter 5

The analysis of Table 5.1 to compare the proportions of males and females in the appendicitis and surgical groups using *OpenEpi* is given in Figure 14.5. The method given in the text corresponds to the Taylor series method. The other methods are discussed in Chapter 9.

Point estimates		Confidence limits	
Type	Value	Lower, Upper	Type
Risk in exposed	8.333%	4.578, 14.44	Taylor series
Risk in unexposed	16.03%	10.66, 23.34	Taylor series
Overall risk	12.17%	8.715, 16.71	Taylor series
Risk ratio	0.5198	0.2612, 1.035	Taylor series
Risk difference	−7.697%	−15.55, 0.1575	Taylor series
Prevented fraction in exposed (pfe)	48.02%	−3.459, 73	

Figure 14.4 Analysis of data from Table 3.2 using OpenEpi.

Odds-based estimates and confidence limits			
Point estimates		Confidence limits	
Type	Value	Lower, Upper	Type
CMLE odds ratio*	1.185	0.7965, 1.774[1]	Mid-*P* exact
		0.7822, 1.808[1]	Fishers exact
Odds ratio	1.185	0.7957, 1.765[1]	Taylor series

Figure 14.5 Analysis of data from Table 7.1 to find an odds ratio using *OpenEpi*.
* Conditional maximum likelihood estimates
[1] 95% confidence interval

```
COMPARISON OF TWO MEANS
Variable      Mean     Variance   Std.Dev.   S.E.Mean  N
Group 1      68.40     271.40      16.47      4.25    15
Group 2      83.42     310.99      17.63      5.09    12
Assuming equal variances, t =    -2.281 with probability = 0.0313 and  25
degrees of freedom
Difference =   -15.02 and Standard Error of difference =     6.58
Confidence interval = (  -28.57,   -1.46)
Assuming unequal variances, t =    -2.264 with probability = 0.0321 and 22.94
degrees of freedom
Difference =   -15.02 and Standard Error of difference =     6.63
Confidence interval = (  -28.74,   -1.29)
F test for equal variances =    1.146, Probability = 0.3983

NOTE: t-tests are two-tailed tests.
```

Figure 14.6 Analysis of data from Table 8.1 to compare two independent means using OpenStat.

Chapter 7

The first example in Chapter 7 compares an observed mean with a population mean. This is easily done in *OpenStat* using "analyses/comparisons/single sample tests". The analysis of the data in Table 7.1, which compares two independent means, is given in Figure 14.6 using *OpenStat*. The program has the option of either entering the means and standard deviations directly, or reading the data from the spreadsheet. In the latter case one must enter two variables, the first corresponding to the transit time for both groups and the second a variable indicating which group the observation belongs to. In this case, the standard deviations in the two groups are similar and so the equal and unequal variance tests give almost the same result. It is common for people to look at the test for equality of variance and depending on whether it is significant or not, to choose either the equal or unequal variance test. The reasoning against this approach is given in the common questions section of Chapter 7 and in general the unequal variance approach is to be preferred.

```
COMPARISON OF TWO MEANS

Variable    Mean      Variance   Std.Dev.   S.E.Mean  N
A              70.17    174.33     13.20       3.81    12
B              76.67    200.79     14.17       4.09    12
Assuming dependent samples, t =   -1.487 with probability = 0.1652 and  11
degrees of freedom
Correlation between A and B =  0.390
Difference =     -6.50 and Standard Error of difference =     4.37
Confidence interval = (  -16.13,    3.13)
t for test of equal variances =   -0.243 with probability = 0.8131

NOTE: t-tests are two-tailed test
```

Figure 14.7 Analysis of data in Table 8.2 to compare two dependent means using OpenStat.

The analysis of the data in Table 7.2 to compare paired observations is shown in Figure 14.7. Here, one has to enter the transit times as two separate columns, with each row corresponding to one person. The test for equal variances is somewhat irrelevant to the analysis, since it is the variance of the differences between the observations that is used, and this is valid even with unequal variances for the two variables. However, if the variances were markedly different, one would think about using a variance stabilizing transformation (Chapter 2).

Chapter 8

Figure 14.8 gives the results of the analysis by *OpenEpi* on the data from a 5 × 2 contingency table given in Table 8.1 using the "Counts/ R × C table" option. The results are the same as those given in the text.

Figure 14.9 gives the results of applying the "Counts/Two by Two" option in *OpenEpi* to the data in Table 8.3 for a 2×2 table. The results give the uncorrected and corrected chi-squared test. They give the one- and two-sided *P*-values, but almost always one should use the two-sided *P*-value. Note that for tables other than 2×2 the two-sided *P*-value is the only one given, since it is difficult to specify a one-sided alternative to the null hypothesis. Figure 14.9 also gives the results of a test known as Fisher's exact test. The calculations of Fisher's exact test are described in earlier editions of this book, but are now omitted because the results are easily available. In essence, Fisher's exact test calculates the probability of the data in the two by two table, under the null hypothesis that the two proportions come from the same population assuming

	Var 2		
	17	5	22
Var 1	25	21	46
	39	34	73
	42	49	91
	32	25	57
	155	134	289

Chi-square for R by C table	
Chi square=	7.146
Degrees of freedom=	4
P-value=	0.1284

Figure 14.8 Analysis of data from Table 9.1 using a chi-squared test with *OpenEpi* R × C table option.

2 × 2 Table statistics			
	Disease		
	(+)	(−)	
(+)	36	14	50
Exposure (−)	30	25	55
	66	39	105

Chi-square and exact measures of association			
Test	Value	*P*-value (1-tail)	*P*-value (2-tail)
Uncorrected chi-square	3.418	0.03225	0.06451
Yates corrected chi-square	2.711	0.04984	0.09969
Fisher's exact		0.04939	0.09879
Mid-*P* exact		0.03454	0.06907

All expected values (row total*column total/grand total) are ⩾5
OK to use chi-square.

Figure 14.9 Analysis of data from Table 9.3 using a chi-squared test to compare two proportions with *OpenEpi* two by two option.

that the margins (totals around the edge of the table) are fixed. The *P*-value is the probability of the observed table and tables more "extreme" (having smaller probability) in either one direction (one tailed) or both directions (two tailed). The mid-*P* method is also described in earlier editions of this book, and halves the

Dose–response analysis					
Stratum 1					
Exposure level	Cases	Controls	Total	Odds of exp.	Odds ratio
0	100	78	178	1.28	1
1	175	173	348	1.01	0.79
2	42	59	101	0.71	0.56
Total	317	310	627		

Mantel–Haenszel summary odds ratios and crude OR for each exposure level

Exposure	MH Summary OR	Crude OR
Level 0 vs. Level 0:	1	1
Level 1 vs. Level 0:	0.789	0.789
Level 2 vs. Level 0:	0.555	0.555

If MH and crude ORs are equal, confounding by the stratifying variable was not present and stratification is unnecessary.

Extended Mantel–Haenszel chi−square for linear trend=	5.68
P-value (1 degree of freedom)=	0.01721

Includes continuity correction. Rosner B. *Fundamentals of Biostatistics*, 5th ed. Duxbury, 2000:606.

Figure 14.10 Analysis of data from Table 9.7 to carry out a chi-squared test for trend using *OpenEpi* counts/dose–response option.

probability of the observed table in calculating the P-value. This is less conservative and has certain theoretical advantages and is the one we advocate. Note that in general (and for this table) the P-values for Fisher's exact test and Yates' corrected chi-squared test agrees and that the mid-P and the uncorrected chi-squared test are also similar.

Figure 14.10 gives the results of applying the "OpenEpi Counts/Dose–response" to the ordinal outcome data in Table 8.6. The result is a chi-squared test with one degree of freedom.

To analyze a matched study, we use the *OpenEpi* "Counts/matched case–control". Figure 14.11 gives the results of applying this to the data of Table 8.7 and the results correspond to those in Chapter 8.

Chapter 9

Figure 14.12 gives the results of the analysis of Table 9.2 on diagnostic tests. It conveniently gives the confidence interval for each measure. The "Wilson Score" method is a more sophisticated method of calculating a confidence interval for a proportion than

Single table analysis				
		Controls		
		(+)	(−)	
	(+)	16	10	26
Cases	(−)	23	5	28
		39	15	54

Measures of association				
			P-values	
Test	Value	d.f.	1-tail	2-tail
McNemar:	5.121	1		0.02364
McNemar with continuity correction:	4.364	1		0.03671
Fisher's exact			0.01754 (P)	0.03508
Mid-P exact			0.01215 (P)	0.02431

There are 33 discordant pairs.
Because this number is ≥ 20, the McNemar test can be used.

Odds-based estimates			
		95% confidence intervals	
Parameter	Point estimate	Lower, Upper	Type
Pair-matched odds ratio:	0.4348	0.207, 0.9134[1]	Taylor series
CMLE odds ratio*	0.4348	0.1981, 0.9012[1]	Mid-*P* exact
		0.1847, 0.9497[1]	Fisher's exact

*Conditional maximum likelihood estimate of odds ratio.
(P) indicates a one-tail *P*-value for protective or negative association; otherwise one-tailed exact *P*-values are for a positive association.
Martin D and Austin H. An efficient program for computing conditional maximum likelihood estimates and exact confidence limits for a common odds ratio. *Epidemiology* 1991; **2**:359–62.

Figure 14.11 Analysis of data from Table 9.10 to compared two matched proportions using a McNemar's test in *OpenEpi* counts/matched case–control option.

the methods described in this book, which is valid for proportions close to 0 or 1. The method is described in Newcombe (1998).[1]

Chapter 10

The Wilcoxon test and the Mann–Whitney U test are available in *OpenStat* under "analysis/non-parametric". Note that for the Wilcoxon test, the paired variables are entered as two columns, whereas in the Mann–Whitney U test the outcome variable is in

	Positive	Negative	Total	
Positive	63	152	215	
Negative	10	740	750	
	73	892	965	

Parameter	Estimate	Lower – Upper 95% CIs	Method
Sensitivity	86.3%	(76.59, 92.39[1])	Wilson score
Specificity	82.96%	(80.35, 85.28[1])	Wilson score
Positive predictive value	29.3%	(23.62, 35.71[1])	Wilson score
Negative predictive value	98.67%	(97.56, 99.27[1])	Wilson score
Diagnostic accuracy	83.21%	(80.72, 85.44[1])	Wilson score
Likelihood ratio of a positive test	5.065	(4.975–5.156)	
Likelihood ratio of a negative test	0.1651	(0.1357–0.201)	

Figure 14.12 Analysis of data from Table 10.2 using OpenEpi "diagnostic or screening test evaluation" option.

one column and a second column indicates which group the subject belongs to. The results of the analysis of the data from Tables 10.1 and 10.2 are given in Figures 14.13a and 14.14a. The output is not very extensive. The P-values are one sided and rely on the Normal approximation, which is less accurate for small samples.

A confidence interval can be obtained using the R commands.

For the paired data:

```
> x1<- c(25,24,28,15,20,23,21,20,20,27)
> x2<-c(18,27,25,20,17,24,24,22,19,19)
>wilcox.test(x1,x2, paired=TRUE, conf.int=TRUE)
```

For the unpaired data:

```
> x1<-c(38,26,29,41,36,31,32,30,35,33)
>x2<-c(45,28,27,38,40,42,39,39,34,45)
>wilcox.test(x1,x2, conf.int=TRUE)
```

The output is given in Figures 14.13b and 14.14b.

Note that R gives the two-sided P-values, and the larger of the sum of the ranks for the Wilcoxon test, whereas *OpenStat* gives one-sided P-values and the smaller of the sum of the ranks.

Chapter 11: Regression and correlation

Figure 11.3 in Chapter 11 is easily reproduced (with the line of best fit) using *OpenStat* "analyses/descriptives x versus y plot". To obtain the regression, we use the "Analyses/Multiple Regression/Block Entry Multiple Regression". The output is given in Figure 14.15 and is somewhat disappointing. The program does not give

```
The Wilcoxon Matched-Pairs Signed-Ranks Test
See pages 75-83 in S. Seigel's Nonparametric Statistics for the
Social Sciences

Ordered cases with cases having 0 differences eliminated:
Number of cases with absolute differences greater than 0 = 10
CASE      before       after    Difference    Signed Rank
  6        23.00       24.00       -1.00          -1.50
  9        20.00       19.00        1.00           1.50
  8        20.00       22.00       -2.00          -3.00
  2        24.00       27.00       -3.00          -5.50
  7        21.00       24.00       -3.00          -5.50
  3        28.00       25.00        3.00           5.50
  5        20.00       17.00        3.00           5.50
  4        15.00       20.00       -5.00          -8.00
  1        25.00       18.00        7.00           9.00
 10        27.00       19.00        8.00          10.00

Smaller sum of ranks (T) =     23.50
Approximately normal z for test statistic T =   0.408
Probability (1-tailed) of greater z =0.3417
NOTE: For N < 25 use tabled values for Wilcoxon Test
```

Figure 14.13a Analysis of data from Table 11.1 using a Wilcoxon test in *OpenStat*.

Wilcoxon signed rank test with continuity correction

data: x1 and x2

V = 31.5, P-value = 0.7193

alternative hypothesis: true location shift is not equal to 0

95 percent confidence interval:

 −2.999967 3.999929

sample estimates:

(pseudo)median

   0.5000412

Figure 14.13b Analysis of data from Table 11.1 using "Wilcoxon test" in *R*.

confidence intervals for the estimates and one has to calculate them from the standard errors as shown in Chapter 11. A number of addition terms need explanation. The beta coefficient is found by first dividing the x variable by its standard deviation, and so the value of 0.846 means that Deadspace increases by 0.846 l for each unit standard deviation increase in height. The adjusted R2 is given by R2(adj) = $1 - (1 - R2)*(n - 2)/(n - k - 1)$, where n is the number of pairs and k the number of independent variables (in this case 1). This allows for the fact that the more independent

```
Mann-Whitney U Test
See pages 116-127 in S. Siegel's Nonparametric Statistics for the
Behavioral Sciences

         Score     Rank       Group
         26.00     1.00         1
         27.00     2.00         2
         28.00     3.00         2
         29.00     4.00         1
         30.00     5.00         1
         31.00     6.00         1
         32.00     7.00         1
         33.00     8.00         1
         34.00     9.00         2
         35.00    10.00         1
         36.00    11.00         1
         38.00    12.50         2
         38.00    12.50         1
         39.00    14.50         2
         39.00    14.50         2
         40.00    16.00         2
         41.00    17.00         1
         42.00    18.00         2
         45.00    19.50         2
         45.00    19.50         2

Sum of Ranks in each Group
Group    Sum     No. in Group
  1      81.50        10
  2     128.50        10

No. of tied rank groups = 3
Statistic U = 26.5000
z Statistic (corrected for ties) = 1.7764, Prob. > z = 0.0378
z test is approximate. Use tables of exact probabilities in
Siegel.
```

Figure 14.14a Analysis of data from Table 11.2 using a Mann–Whitney *U* test in *OpenStat*.

```
Wilcoxon rank sum test with continuity correction

data: x1 and x2
W = 26.5, P-value = 0.08175
alternative hypothesis: true location shift is not equal to 0
95 percent confidence interval:
 -10.000052  1.000023
sample estimates:
difference in location
      -5.415387
```

Figure 14.14b Analysis of data from Table 11.2 using "Wilcoxon test" in *R*.

```
Linear Regression

Dependent variable: Deadspace

Variable      Beta      B          Std.Err.  t        Prob.>t  VIF    TOL
  Height      0.846     1.033      0.180     5.728    0.000    1.000  1.000
Intercept     0.000    -82.485     26.301   -3.136    0.008

SOURCE        DF        SS         MS        F        Prob.>F
Regression    1         5607.432   5607.432  32.814   0.0001
Residual      13        2221.502   170.885
Total         14        7828.933

R2 = 0.7162, F = 32.81, D.F. = 1 13, Prob>F = 0.0001
Adjusted R2 = 0.6944

Standard Error of Estimate = 13.07
F = 32.814 with probability = 0.000
Block 1 met entry requirements
```

Figure 14.15 Analysis of linear regression data from Table 12.2 using *OpenStat*.

```
Total Expected Events for Experimental Group =   11.375
Observed Events for Experimental Group =   10.000
Total Expected Events for Control Group =   10.625
Observed Events for Control Group =   12.000
Chisquare =    0.344 with probability = 0.442
Risk =    0.778, Log Risk =   -0.250, Std.Err. Log Risk =   0.427
95 Percent Confidence interval for Log Risk = (-1.087,0.586)
95 Percent Confidence interval for Risk = (0.337,1.796)
```

Figure 14.16 Analysis of survival data from Table 13.3 using *OpenStat*.

variables are in the model, the better the fit (until with *n* independent variables we can get a perfect fit), and so we need to trade off the goodness of fit with the number of independent variables. There is an option to save the residuals and the fitted values, and these can be used to check assumptions such as the Normality of the residuals (by eye) and constant variance. The use and interpretation of multiple regression with more than one independent variable is described in *Statistics at Square Two*.

Chapter 12: Survival analysis

The Kaplan–Meier curves shown in Chapter 12 (Figure 12.1) can be obtained from *OpenStat* through "analyses/non-parametric/ Kaplan–Meier survival". The events must be coded 1 for an event and 2 for a censored observation, and the survival times must be integers. The results are shown in Figure 14.16 and are the same as given in Chapter 12. There is also an option to plot the two survival curves.

Reference

1. Newcombe RG. Interval estimation for the difference between independent proportions: comparison of eleven methods. *Statistics in Medicine* 1998;**17**:873–90.

Websites

Chi	www.sheffield.ac.uk/scharr/sections/hsr/statistics/staff/campbell.html
OpenStat	statpages.org/miller/OpenStat
OpenEpi	www.OpenEpi.com
OpenOffice	openoffice.org-site.com
R	www.r-project.org
SISA	www.quantitativeskills.com/sisa
Stata	www.stata.com
Xycoon	http://www.xycoon.com/index.htm

Answers to exercises

1.1 Median 0.71, range 0.10 to 1.24, first quartile 0.535, third quartile 0.84 μmol/24 h. The only values that change, in each case, are the range.

1.2 Continuous, ordinal, count, categorical.

2.1 Mean = 2.41, SD = 1.27. No, because the mean is less than 2 SDs and data are positive.

2.2 Mean = 0.697 μmol/24 h, SD = 0.2410 μmol/24 h, approx. 95% range 0.215 to 1.179 μmol/l. Points excluded are 0.10 and 1.24. 2/40 or 5%. Mean changes to 0.722 and SD to 0.333.

2.3 (a) Data distribution is quite symmetric, so display summary as mean ± SD. (b) The data distribution is skewed, so display summary as a box-whisker plot. (c) The data are categorical so use a bar chart.

3.1 (a) False, the statement says nothing about actual risks of benefits. (b) False, the statement says nothing about what is known as "power" (see Chapter 6). (c) False, this is the absolute risk reduction. (d) True.

3.2 (a) True, (b) False, it is around 50, (c) True.

3.3 (a) True, (b) True.

3.4 20%.

3.5 5.

3.6 Relative risk 1.79, odds ratio 2.09.

4.1 SE (mean) = 0.074 μmol/24 h.

4.2 A uniform or flat distribution. Population mean 4.5, since symmetric about (0–9).

4.3 The distribution will be approximately Normal, mean 4.5, and SD $2.87/\sqrt{5} = 1.28$.

5.1 The reference range is 12.26–57.74, and so the observed value of 52 is included in it.

5.2 95% CI 32.73 to 37.27.

5.3 Difference in means, = 1.3 g/dl, SE 0.422, 95% CI 0.48 to 2.12 g/dl.

5.4 SE (percentage) = 2.1%, SE (difference) = 3.7%, difference = 3.4%. 95% CI 3.9% to 10.7%.

5.5 Difference in proportions 0.193, 95% CI 0.033 to 0.348.
5.6 OR = 4.89, 95% CI 4.00 to 5.99.

6.1 (a) False (this is a common mistake!), (b) true, (c) false (this is the observed difference), (d) false, (e) false.
6.2 (a) True, (b) true, (c) false (see reference 3 in Chapter 5), (d) false (can't say this is important without more data), (e) false.
6.3 $z = 1.3/0.422 = 3.1$, $P \approx 0.0027$. (Appendix A)

7.1 95% CI = 37.5 to 40.5 KA units.
7.2 $t = 2.652$, d.f. = 17, 2. $P = 0.017$.
7.3 0.56 g/dl, $t = 1.243$, d.f. = 20, $P = 0.23$, 95% CI -0.38 to 1.50 g/dl.
7.4 15 days, $t = 1.758$, d.f. = 9, $P = 0.11$, 95% CI -4.30 to 34.30 days.

8.1 Standard $X^2 = 3.295$, d.f. = 4, $P = 0.51$. Trend $X^2 = 2.25$, d.f. = 1, $P = 0.13$.
8.2 $X^2 = 3.916$, d.f. = 1, $P = 0.048$, difference in rates 9%, 95% CI 0.3% to 17.9%.
8.3 $X^2 = 0.931$, d.f. = 1, $P = 0.33$, difference in rates 15%, 95% CI -7.7% to 38%.
8.4 $X^2 = 8.949$, d.f. = 3, $P = 0.03$. Yes, practice C; if this is omitted the remaining practices give $X^2 = 0.241$, d.f. = 2, $P = 0.89$. (Both χ^2 tests by quick method.)
8.5 $X^2 = 5.685$, d.f. = 1, $P = 0.017$. This is statistically significant and the CI in Exercise 5.5 does not include zero.
8.6 $X^2 = 285.96$, d.f. = 1, $P < 0.001$. Highly significant and CI in Exercise 5.6 is a long way from 1.
8.7 X2 5 0.6995, d.f. 5 1, P 5 0.40. The z value was 0.84 and from Table A (Appendix) we find $0.37 < P < 0.42$. Note $z^2 = X^2$.
8.8 Using McNemar's test $X^2 = (|28 - 13|-1)^2/(28 + 13) = 4.78$, $P = 0.029$.

9.1 Draw up 2 × 2 table

		Disease		
		Present	**Absent**	**Total**
Test	Positive	10	500	510
	Negative	0	9490	
	Total	10	9990	10 000

From the fact that the prevalence is 1 in 1000, we have 10 people with the disease. Since sensitivity is 100% that means in those with the disease, all have a positive test. In those without the disease $0.95 \times 9990 = 9490$ will have a negative result. This means that 500 will be positive. This means that $10/510 = 2\%$ will have disease given positive result.

9.2 Odds of having disease is $0.03/0.97$. Thus odds after disease are $0.97 \times 0.15 = 0.45$. This probability $= 0.45/(1 + 0.45) = 0.31$.

9.3 (a) False (sensitivity is a property of the test), (b) false (sensitivity versus 1–specificity), (c) true.(d) true.

10.1 Smaller total $= -24$. Not significant.

10.2 Mann-Whitney statistic $= 74$. The group on the new remedy. No.

11.1 $r = -0.848$.

11.2 $r_s = -0.868$.

11.3 $y = 36.1 - 2.34x$. This means that, on average, for every 1 mile increase in mean distance the attendance rate drops by 2.34%. This can be safely accepted only within the area measured here.

11.4 SE $= 0.39, 95\%$ CI $-2.34 - 2.145 \times 0.39$ to $-2.34 + 2.145 \times 0.39 = -3.2\%$ to -1.5%.

11.5 $r = -0.772, r_s = -0.870, y = 31.3 - 1.48x$. Thus Spearman's rank little changed but Pearson and slope affected. $r = -0.800, r_s = -0.820, y = 34.93 - 2.22x$, less effect.

12.1 $O_A = 6, E_A = 8.06, O_B = 8, E_B = 5.94$. Log rank $X^2 = 1.31$, d.f. $= 1, P = 0.25$. No Change results from changing the survival times, which shows that the main driver for the log rank test is the number of events.

12.2 Risk $= 0.55, 95\%$ CI 0.19 to 1.60.

13.1 Matched case–control study.

13.2 Cohort study.

13.3 Cross-sectional study.

13.4 Randomized controlled trial.

13.5 Quasi-experimental design.

Glossary of statistical terms

(An online glossary is given at www.stats.gla.ac.uk/steps/glossary/)

Alternative hypothesis In hypothesis testing, this hypothesis will be "accepted" when the null hypothesis is rejected. In a clinical trial, it may a difference in treatments that would make it worth changing treatments.

ARR – absolute risk reduction The difference in rates of an outcome event between the control and experimental groups.

Bar chart A chart showing the frequencies of the values of a categorical variable. The bars are generally separated, and their lengths are proportional to the counts in the categories.

Baseline measure A measure of some characteristic that is recorded for subjects at the start of a study, before any treatment commences.

Bayesian methods Methods which allow parameters to have distributions. Initially the parameter θ is assigned a prior distribution $P(\theta)$, and after data, X, have been collected a posterior distribution $P(\theta|X)$ is obtained using *Bayes' theorem*, which links the two via the *likelihood* $p(X|\theta)$.

Bias A systematic error that leads to results which are consistently either too large or too small.

Binary A binary categorical variable can take one of two values (e.g. true/false or male/female). Sometimes referred to as a dichotomous variable.

Bonferroni correction A method of correcting for n multiple comparisons by only rejecting the null hypothesis if P is less than α/n where α is the significance level.

Box–whisker plot A chart that is often used to compare two or more samples of ordinal or continuous variables. A boxplot shows the median, lower and upper quartiles, the interquartile range, the maximum and minimum values, and possible outliers.

Case–control study An observational study designed to find relationships between, for example, a risk factor and a disease. A group of cases (with the disease) are compared with a group of controls (without the disease) with regard to their exposure to the risk factor. The data are summarized by an odds ratio.

Censored Censored data often occur in studies of survival data. The data are censored if the event (e.g. death or recurrence of disease) has not been observed during the duration of the study.

Census A survey of an entire population.

Central limit theorem A theorem which tells you about the distribution of the sample mean of large samples. For large samples, the sample mean is Normally distributed.

Cohort A group of subjects who share some characteristic in common, which are followed up over time.

Confidence interval A range of values that are believed, with a particular probability, to contain the true parameter value. A 95% confidence interval, for example, implies that, were the estimation process repeated again and again, then 95% of the calculated intervals would be expected to contain the true parameter value. Note that the stated probability refers to properties of the interval and not to the parameter itself, which is not considered a random variable.

Confounding The effects of two variables are said to be confounded if they are inseparable. For example, in a clinical trial, if all men were on one treatment and all women on another then gender and treatment would be confounded.

Continuous A variable is continuous if it can take any value in a particular range (i.e. it can take decimal values), for example height, weight, and blood pressure.

Control group A group of subjects used in a study as a comparison with the group of primary interest.

Correlation The correlation coefficient is a measure of the degree of linear association between two continuous variables. A value of +1 indicates perfect positive association, a value of −1 indicates perfect negative association, and a value of 0 indicates no linear association. The value is highly sensitive to a few abnormal data values.

Cross-sectional study An observational study in which subjects are investigated as one point in time.

Crossover trial One in which subjects receive more than one treatment in sequential order.

Data dredging The highly undesirable practice of searching through data in an attempt to find an interesting result. It is sometimes called data fishing.

Dependent variable A somewhat confusing term that is used in statistical modeling. When one variable is believed to influence another variable, the latter is called the dependent variable. It is sometimes called a response or outcome variable, and is plotted on the vertical axis of a graph.

Dichotomous Taking two possible values (i.e. binary).

Discrete A variable is discrete if it can take only certain values. These are usually whole numbers (e.g. counts, such as the number of visits to the GP).

Distribution Distributions describe the histograms of whole populations. There are several distributions that are commonly used (e.g. the normal distribution).

Double-blind A trial is double-blind if neither the subject nor the person conducting the assessment of the subject knows to which treatment group the subject has been allocated. Uses of the term vary.

Equivalence study A study in which the objective is to show that two treatments are equivalent in outcome, as opposed to showing that one is superior to the other. The two types of study need to be designed differently.

Estimate A value calculated from a sample when you are really interested in the value for the population. It is an informed guess.

Experiment A comparative study in which the researchers are able to control the factor of interest. A typical example is a clinical trial in which one treatment is given to one group of subjects and another treatment is given to a second group of subjects. The researchers determine who receives which treatment.

Factor A variable with (a few) discrete levels. The term is also used to describe a condition controlled by a researcher in an experiment (e.g. different treatments).

Geometric mean A type of average, usually close to the median. It is related to the product of all the data values. It occurs when positively skewed data have been transformed by taking logs before analysis.

Hazard A form of risk used in survival analysis. It is the risk of an event at a point in time, *conditional* on the subject surviving to that point in time.

Histogram A chart that is used to represent continuous data. It consists of bars which are adjacent, and whose area is proportional to the frequency for that range of values.

Incidence Proportion of people, initially clear of a disease, who develop it over a given time period. It is a *rate* and is often equated to a *risk*.

Independence Two events are said to be independent if knowing about one tells you nothing about the other.

Independent variable In a regression model, the variable that predicts the *dependent* variable. Note that a model can have more than one independent variable and they need not be independent of each other.

Intention-to-treat analysis In clinical trials subjects may drop out of the study or change treatment groups. An intention-to-treat analysis retains data from all subjects in the group to which they were originally allocated. This is considered to be the correct way to deal with dropouts.

Interaction An interaction exists between two variables or factors if the effect of one depends on the value of the other.

Interquartile range The difference between the lower and upper quartiles, which includes the central 50% of the data, used to describe the variability in ordinal or skewed data.

Likert-type scale A scale on questionnaires where a subject is asked to what extent they agree with a statement. It usually contains five or seven categories.

Linear association A linear association exists between two continuous variables if a reasonable amount of variability in one is explained by a straight-line equation with the other. The scatterplot with show points scattered around a straight line.

Longitudinal study A study in which subjects are followed over time. Characteristics are measured at several points in time.

Mean An average value that is computed by adding together all of the values and dividing by the number of values.

Measure of dispersion Parameter describing the width or spread of a distribution for quantitative data (e.g. standard deviation or variance).

Measure of location Parameter describing the center of a distribution for quantitative data (e.g. mean and median).

Median The middle value in a set of data. It is most often used when describing skewed data.

Mode The most frequently occurring value, used to describe nominal or ordinal data.

Model An equation which relates two or more variables.

Multiple testing The rather dangerous practice of performing several tests on the same set of data. This is particularly undesirable if the tests are thought of after the data have been collected.

Mutually exclusive Two events are mutually exclusive if both cannot occur together.

Negative predictive value In diagnostic testing, the probability that you do not have the disease when the test is negative. The value of the negative prediction rate can be affected by the prevalence rate.

Nominal A categorical variable is nominal if it can take a set of values that are not ordered (e.g. ethnic origin).

Non-parametric test A test which requires no distributional assumptions about the data. Note the test itself is non-parametric, not the data!

Normal distribution A symmetrical bell-shaped distribution that is often used to model data. For a Normal distribution the mean and the median will coincide. About 95% of the data from a Normal distribution will lie within plus or minus two standard deviations from the mean.

Null hypothesis The hypothesis that states that there is no effect or difference. We assume that this hypothesis is true, and it is only rejected if there is a weight of evidence against it.

Number needed to treat The inverse of the absolute risk reduction. The number of patients one would need to treat to get one *extra* event compared to the control treatment.

Observational study A non-experimental study in which subjects are observed. Examples include cohort and case–control studies.

Odds The ratio of the probability an event will happen to the probability of it not happening.

Odds ratio A ratio of odds in two groups, often used in case–control studies as an approximation to estimating the relative risk.

One-sided test A test in which the alternative hypothesis is that an effect or difference is in a particular direction (e.g. greater than zero). If one intends to use a one-sided test, one should state this at the design stage and have very good reason to do so.

Ordinal Categorical data in which the various values have a natural order.

Outlier A value in a data set which appears to be a long way from the rest of the data. It may be an error or an unusual or interesting value.

Parameter A characteristic of a *population* such as a population mean or standard deviation. It is also used as the name of the coefficients in a regression model.

Parametric test A statistical test which relies on the data having a particular distribution (often the Normal distribution).

Percentile The value below which a particular percentage of the data lie, for example 25% of observations will lie below the 25th percentile. Note that the median is also the 50th centile.

Pie chart A circle that is divided into sections so that the area of each slice is proportional to the number represented. It is used when all subdivisions of the subject are being studied, and you want to show how the relative sizes of the subdivisions differ. Three-dimensional pie charts can be very misleading.

Pilot study A small-scale study that is conducted in order to investigate the usefulness of some method or tool (e.g. a questionnaire) that you intend to use in the full-scale study.

Placebo An inert substance, indistinguishable from the active drug, which is given to the control group. This enables both subjects and researchers to remain blinded to the treatment allocation.

Population The entire set of subjects or items about which you want information.

Population parameter Characteristic of a population that you are trying to estimate.

Positive predictive value In diagnostic testing, the probability that you do have the disease when the test is positive. The value can be affected by the prevalence rate.

Power The probability that you will find a statistically significant difference using a statistical test when that size of difference actually exists. See *type II error*.

Predictor variable Sometimes called an explanatory variable or (rather confusingly) *independent variable*. The variable that is plotted on the horizontal axis, and that is used in modeling to predict the values of the response variable.

Prevalence The proportion of subjects with a characteristic at one point in time (contrast with *incidence*).

Probability A measure of how likely an event is. All probabilities range between 0 and 1; a value of +1 denotes an event is certain to happen and 0 denotes an event is never going to happen.

Prospective cohort study A study in which a group of subjects is followed forward in time. Usually the level of risk is measured first, and the subjects are monitored for development of a disease.

P-value The probability of observing a test statistic at least as extreme as that actually observed *if the null hypothesis were true*. A small *P*-value is interpreted as strong evidence against the null hypothesis. Confidence intervals are more informative than *P*-values.

Qualitative data Observations or information characterized by measurement on a categorical scale.

Quantitative data Data in numerical quantities, such as continuous measurements or counts.

Quartiles Points which divide the data into four quarters. There are three quartiles, lower, median, and upper. Note that they are points not areas, so an observation can be above the upper quartile, not in the upper quartile.

Random sample A sample chosen from the population by chance—each member has an equal chance of being selected.

Randomization The method of allocation of treatments to subjects using the principle of chance.

Randomized controlled trial (RCT) A study in which at least two treatment groups are studied, one of which is a control group. Randomization is used to allocate the subjects to the treatment groups.

Range The smallest and the largest values in the data. In statistics it is not common to give the range as the difference between the two.

Rate The proportion of subjects who develop a disease over a period of time. To avoid decimals it is usually expressed as a portion of a large number, such as deaths per thousand per year.

Regression line A straight-line equation that is used to model the relationship between a response variable and one or more predictor variables.

Relative risk (RR) The ratio of the risk of some event in one group relative to that in another group.

Repeated-measures study A study of subjects where more than one measure is taken on the same subject, usually over a period of time. Measures on the same subject will be associated or correlated, so special measures of analysis are needed.

Response variable Sometimes called the outcome variable or the dependent variable. In plots it will be represented on the vertical axis. In modeling it is the variable being predicted by the model.

Retrospective study An observational study in which subjects are chosen by disease status and then followed back in time in order to ascertain their exposure to a risk. Typically it is a case–control study.

RRR – relative risk reduction The proportion of the original risk that was eliminated by a treatment. 1–RR.

Risk Probability of an event happening in a given period of time.

Sample A set of people or items chosen for study from a population.

Sampling frame The list of the entire population of interest used to draw a sample.

Scatterplot A graph showing the relationship between two continuous variables. Each symbol on the graph is determined by the pair of values of the variables.

Sensitivity For a diagnostic test, the percentage of people with the disease who will test positive.

Significance level The probability of rejecting the null hypothesis when it is in fact true. A level of 5% is usually chosen. Sometimes known as the type I error rate.

Single-blind A study in which the subjects are unaware of which treatment they are receiving. However, usage of the term is inconsistent. Some people use the term to refer to studies where the assessor, but not the subjects, are unaware of the treatment allocation.

Skewness Data are skewed if the histogram has a long tail on one side. A positive skew is a long tail to the right and a negative skew a long tail to the left.

SnNout If a test has a high sensitivity, a negative result rules a diagnosis out.

Specificity For a diagnostic test, the percentage of people without the disease who will test negative.

SpPin If a test has a high specificity, a positive result rules a diagnosis in.

Standard deviation A measure of spread or variability, mainly used for continuous symmetrical data in conjunction with the mean.

Standard error A measure of the uncertainty in an estimate from a sample. Strictly speaking it is the *standard deviation* of the sampling distribution of a statistic (mean, mean difference, proportion, difference in proportions).

Statistic A value calculated from a sample (e.g. the sample mean and sample proportion).

Survey An observational study that is used to find out the characteristics of a population. The method of sampling is critically important.

Survival data Data that arise from studies where the outcome of interest is the time until a particular event (often death). Censored data are often obtained from such a study.

Test statistic A statistic that is calculated from a sample and used in a statistical test. A "large" or extreme value of a test statistic will result in a low P-value and thus rejection of the null hypothesis.

Transformation If data are not Normally distributed, they are sometimes transformed on to a different scale by a mathematical manipulation. Common transformations are the natural logarithm, square root, and reciprocal.

Treatment group A group in a study that receives an active treatment which is under investigation.

Two-sided test A test where the alternative hypothesis is that the effect of interest can be in either direction (e.g. where a drug can be worse or better than placebo).

Type I error Rejecting the null hypothesis when it is true (i.e. claiming to have found an effect that is not really there. The Type I error rate is usually denoted by the Greek letter alpha, α.

Type II error Failing to reject the null hypothesis when it is false (i.e. not finding an effect even though it is there). The Type II error rate is usually denoted by the Greek letter beta, β.

One minus the type II error, i.e. $1 - \beta$ is usually referred to as the *power*.

Variable A characteristic, subject to variability, that can be measured.

Variance The value of the *standard deviation* squared. The units of variance are the original units of measurement squared. The *standard deviation* is much easier to understand, since it is measured in the original units of the data.

Appendix

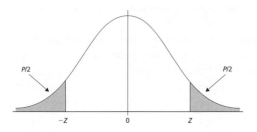

Table A Probabilities related to multiples of standard deviations for a normal distribution.

Number of standard deviations (z)	Probability of getting an observation at least as far from the mean (two-sided P)
0 · 0	1 · 00
0 · 1	0 · 92
0 · 2	0 · 84
0 · 3	0 · 76
0 · 4	0 · 69
0 · 5	0 · 62
0 · 6	0 · 55
0 · 674	0 · 500
0 · 7	0 · 48
0 · 8	0 · 42
0 · 9	0 · 37
1 · 0	0 · 31
1 · 1	0 · 27
1 · 2	0 · 23
1 · 3	0 · 19
1 · 4	0 · 16
1 · 5	0 · 13
1 · 6	0 · 11
1 · 645	0 · 100
1 · 7	0 · 089
1 · 8	0 · 072
1 · 9	0 · 057
1 · 96	0 · 050
2 · 0	0 · 045
2 · 1	0 · 036
2 · 2	0 · 028
2 · 3	0 · 021
2 · 4	0 · 016
2 · 5	0 · 012
2 · 576	0 · 010
3 · 0	0 · 0027
3 · 291	0 · 0010

Table B Random numbers.

```
35368 65415 14425 97294 44734 54870 84495 39332 72708 52000 02219 86130 30264 56203 26518
93023 53965 19527 72819 42973 38037 37056 13200 09831 41367 40828 25938 05655 99010 88115
92226 65530 10966 29733 73902 19009 74733 68041 83166 92796 64846 79200 38776 09312 72234
15542 85361 44069 61445 82994 45169 79458 52221 37132 67125 62700 83475 99850 31670 50750
96424 65745 74877 48473 54281 67837 11167 74898 83136 10498 10660 65810 16373 80382 21874
17946 97751 54049 83077 03256 51947 88278 23891 53495 07101 95811 73035 83017 18532 59650
71495 36712 01513 30802 47228 52799 97961 82519 22756 69151 09052 38681 38858 38807 02422
16762 98574 78301 62647 29247 22936 62778 56694 70597 48880 33162 76138 97425 78283 42063
37969 66660 77823 54923 75832 99974 13868 94446 99521 44775 76649 00502 73424 21068 87880
25471 88920 39906 81436 70910 02631 93238 41952 87493 33559 64733 24688 78583 31506 24845
68507 79643 15204 84794 60093 29874 61851 05751 21960 70131 42137 73723 19252 23912 77751
67385 88293 46249 53036 47309 68803 15155 28222 06764 92367 25490 18494 42546 75268 05988
58948 40572 79817 40486 40494 20843 07388 74732 71655 17445 28489 84528 93922 67324 59120
70476 23299 17965 93629 28988 82399 81811 86373 91600 99962 28784 77326 24912 81992 66011
72887 41730 95940 54210 58480 96724 41954 91803 43078 85644 50014 93038 56037 79787 10707
70205 26256 91417 78629 16268 47156 32065 54588 74250 24739 04128 53966 74106 70159 80428
78883 36361 28182 51842 61426 27799 75951 58854 77236 04606 26949 56428 28495 41766 50059
89970 55101 66660 36953 02774 45020 54988 19226 44811 96941 70693 68847 07633 22289 94290
34382 04274 02116 37857 72075 90908 56584 67907 15075 63216 49006 24748 34289 55142 91206
16999 91140 64818 23018 09217 46068 32467 63844 72589 35456 44840 90800 50692 33298 74323
16329 39676 37510 35590 45888 77371 58301 79434 17500 48320 08953 18242 15133 24137 07323
31983 83436 93006 12640 00403 91457 62602 12245 27670 61492 89166 69421 79505 47104 50817
92780 80153 81458 82215 71536 03586 44007 85679 68186 85375 15373 57441 10034 74455 18466
70834 75678 78777 79731 06046 02386 18059 89623 65480 69345 49447 10358 74307 68861 87853
10100 85365 77687 36241 87563 06298 81828 40194 30647 36237 17793 50680 63701 39522 86006
84265 60501 17148 13657 40775 64773 62103 16356 99405 08598 81881 62732 36765 11895 63933
74041 62109 30831 62133 29462 30144 62081 79158 09737 72614 74806 25554 50911 43289 30344
02882 45141 58967 19688 48208 65679 18296 19080 03529 46017 33799 45518 31075 39740 93387
67647 56443 57816 49471 23525 76582 30085 90312 07397 42747 04242 58569 80087 45598 34374
99668 68326 47357 94812 65654 01097 55260 80990 46748 06416 93919 64520 54666 82278 59328
12013 30983 00370 40243 44457 18279 69740 39061 00548 21321 11249 48478 14917 26056 89506
55581 69068 66561 75671 07363 22939 93007 45319 48358 27534 60873 51076 20823 28185 49038
74957 53949 40414 15035 90232 28946 78073 75923 43081 16030 32935 30947 64395 03271 21345
65073 60950 92314 02037 82817 33518 49680 20095 51301 91889 78488 75298 29067 11355 69994
05110 83292 51335 64460 37648 72915 99688 62628 41297 36039 04436 82738 76614 55630 35803
54053 98104 12386 15646 89759 55889 14513 96192 19957 06186 40853 38011 97401 04047 66722
52351 72086 70257 83693 62924 79060 79683 03143 10627 45371 78404 50185 67515 65094 91111
10759 18901 07590 07727 37140 95782 41994 71688 72341 73665 66833 14138 20949 91852 42847
67322 87517 27043 12936 81043 27338 81679 88420 28220 65441 55517 96640 60178 84161 64239
37634 07842 34936 26836 48230 52786 01114 61335 39149 34268 70089 93491 91616 22522 06577
90556 62996 52252 42541 12781 40917 41661 96994 88818 93137 45130 34502 40479 65832 79294
07067 12854 23166 49012 56479 22674 69603 47846 91920 19188 94206 30370 50741 79932 88916
82945 28472 46267 45857 67101 39905 25753 75462 87523 01394 10135 26758 88652 34480 37901
33399 81517 64127 82407 23689 46598 23814 89327 87057 67715 30785 58496 38661 23259 19631
51428 25572 62696 33117 66242 11735 68466 90598 30201 25770 96006 48256 60967 49546 74989
45246 23347 48896 15828 69240 93948 27855 21999 19155 72859 78754 40094 39323 37570 73953
24384 49141 78464 73448 78883 25730 24813 36087 47883 50473 38354 25620 08787 61463 95219
43550 53461 42673 12646 87988 01411 58160 76833 53423 45490 23316 84940 81917 52712 10575
67691 02660 28326 46648 00840 02753 12403 29024 03017 28175 23557 64382 71324 17581 63090
49360 13426 04763 85671 40498 18689 99523 50400 00562 02112 00219 84376 42585 90350 96349
42432 49348 10219 99564 70165 82692 85914 81874 60401 37323 80781 59989 00844 82734 60942
68547 85157 26956 52508 10019 18964 03084 21624 95686 76579 53032 44148 74984 81609 42544
26081 21040 57032 30827 61940 50305 13410 22158 91529 35888 48318 13355 12491 31827 31256
16113 01090 72822 51906 23547 06985 93466 74652 33329 18298 75319 55988 76412 47573 49236
88368 50633 62276 50244 14896 21158 49633 92045 25400 49228 20287 69106 32732 88075 20196
37861 95795 39254 87408 16929 87171 38600 61330 80663 56488 43425 08589 53842 39410 55751
```

Index

Note: Page numbers in **bold** type refer to figures; those in italic refer to tables or boxed material.